Clinical Decision Making and Judgement in Nursing

For Churchill Livingstone:

Senior Commissioning Editor: Jacqueline Curthoys
Project Development Manager: Karen Gilmour
Project Manager: Gail Murray
Designer: Judith Wright

Clinical Decision Making and Judgement in Nursing

Edited by

Carl Thompson BSc(Hons) PhD RN
Research Fellow and Head of Graduate School, Centre for Evidence-based Nursing, Department of Health Studies, University of York, York, UK

Dawn Dowding BSc(Hons) PhD RGN
Programme Leader, Nursing Research Initiative for Scotland, University of Stirling, Stirling, UK

Foreword by

Sarah Mullally
Chief Nursing Officer, Department of Health, London, UK

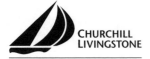
CHURCHILL
LIVINGSTONE

EDINBURGH LONDON OXFORD NEW YORK PHILADELPHIA ST LOUIS SYDNEY TORONTO 2002

CHURCHILL LIVINGSTONE
An imprint of Elsevier Science Limited

First published 2002
Reprinted 2002

SMC   610.73 THO

ISBN 0 443 07076 8

British Library Cataloguing in Publication Data
A catalogue record for this book is available from the British Library

Library of Congress Cataloging in Publication Data
A catalog record for this book is available from the Library of Congress

Note
Medical knowledge is constantly changing. As new information
becomes available, changes in treatment, procedures, equipment and
the use of drugs become necessary. The editors, contributors and the
publishers have taken care to ensure that the information given in
this text is accurate and up to date. However, readers are strongly
advised to confirm that the information, especially with regard to drug
usage, complies with the latest legislation and standards of practice.

 your source for books,
journals and multimedia
in the health sciences
www.elsevierhealth.com

The
publisher's
policy is to use
**paper manufactured
from sustainable forests**

Printed in China
C/02

Contents

Contributors

Jane Cioffi RN BAppSc(AdvNsg) GradDipEd(Nsg) MAppSc(Nsg) PhD
School of Nursing, Family and Community Health,
University of Western Sydney, Richmond, Australia

Robert Crouch PhD RN FRCN
Consultant Nurse/Senior Lecturer, Emergency Department,
Southampton General Hospital and School of Nursing and Midwifery,
University of Southampton, Southampton, UK

Dawn Dowding BSc(Hons) PhD RGN
Programme Leader, Nursing Research Initiative for Scotland,
University of Stirling, Stirling, UK

Mark Fenton MA RMN
Research Nurse, Cochrane Schizophrenia Group, Oxford, UK

Kate Flemming BSc(Hons) MSc RGN
Lecturer in Evidence based Nursing, Department of Health Studies,
University of York, York, UK

Dorothy McCaughan BA MSc RGN
Research Fellow, Centre for Evidence based Nursing,
Department of Health Studies, University of York, York, UK

Maxine Offredy BA(Hons) MPhil PGCE RN HV
Senior Lecturer, Faculty of Health and Human Sciences,
University of Hertfordshire, Hatfield, UK

Jo Rycroft-Malone MSc BSc(Hons) RN
R&D Fellow, RCN Institute, Radcliffe Infirmary, Oxford, UK

Carl Thompson BSc(Hons) PhD RN
Research Fellow and Head of Graduate School,
Centre for Evidence based Nursing, Department of Health Studies,
University of York, York, UK

Foreword

All nurses make clinical decisions. They make judgements about the needs of patients in their care and decisions about what interventions are required.

Experienced nurses claim that this is a tacit process that draws on acquired knowledge and professional experience. Exercising professional expertise in this way may be an essential and natural feature of everyday nursing practice, but there is a risk that implicit judgements and decisions will elude the scrutiny and challenge that form a necessary condition for accountable professional practice.

It is right that as nurses we are exhorted to base our professional practice on sound evidence and to be open and transparent about our judgements and decisions. We must be able to explain and to justify what we propose and what we do because we claim to act in the interests of others. But being able to weigh up the relative merits of evidence from a number of sources and to apply a systematic approach to determine conclusions upon which to propose an appropriate course of action are acquired skills. Learning to reason is as much a professional competency as knowing the facts about a disease or a particular technique for delivering care.

Carl Thompson, Dawn Dowding and the other contributors to this book have done an excellent job in marshalling and explaining the theories and practicalities of professional reasoning in nursing. They have made complex theories both accessible and relevant to everyday professional practice. This book will help nurses to think hard about how they make clinical decisions, how they use evidence to inform that process and what techniques and support can enhance their reasoning. In short, it will help them to become more accountable.

In any human activity such as nursing there is always a risk of errors of judgement of faulty reasoning. We have a professional obligation to reduce this risk to the absolute minimum and to try to ensure that clinical decision making is explicable and defensible. This book is a significant contribution to the literature and has the potential to help nurses to do just that.

Sarah Mullally

1

Decision making and judgement in nursing – an introduction

Carl Thompson   *Dawn Dowding*

No sensible decision can be made any longer without taking into account not only the world as it is, but the world as it will be. ...
Isaac Asimov (1920–92)

KEY ISSUES

◆ Healthcare decision making is associated with uncertainty and health care professionals have to deal with this uncertainty in their decision making.

◆ Key policy drivers have led to the development of an evidence based culture in health care with a focus on the quality of decisions taken by health care professionals.

◆ Judgements and decision making are intricately linked and one cannot be examined without an understanding of the other.

◆ This book examines a number of normative (how decisions should be made in an ideal world), descriptive (how decisions are made in the real world) and prescriptive (how decisions can be improved in the real world) theories and applications.

◆ Intuition and expertise are important factors in decision making and judgement in nursing but cannot be relied upon as a successful solo strategy for good decision making.

WHY WRITE THIS BOOK?

Who could dispute that nurses and midwives make sensible decisions? The quote from Asimov that starts this book might, indeed should, raise some interesting questions in the mind of the reader. One question that arises is 'If a decision is to be considered sensible then surely some knowledge of what the future might look like after the decision is made is required?'. We can apply this question to nursing decisions and at this point suddenly some of the decisions we make as nurses and midwives may not look quite so sensible. How many of us can truthfully say that we know what the future (even in the short term) is going to look like? How many of us have thought something (predictable) is going to happen, only to have something unexpected take its place? Of course, people predict the future when making decisions all the time, otherwise choices would be made with no thought as to the likely consequences of our actions. When making choices we draw on a variety of sources of information: experience, the 'first principles' of stored knowledge or facts, the expertise of others, and occasionally we may look at the experiences of tens, hundreds, even thousands, of others in the form of research evidence.

Of course, such prediction is fallible and flawed. Our experiences can be distorted with hindsight, people can be selective in telling us the information they think we need, first principles often have to be recast as new knowledge replaces old (e.g. giving concentrated oxygen to neonatal babies was considered a good course of action for many years – it was later found to cause blindness) and research can be flawed, often appearing to warrant the services of a translator just to make it understandable. Moreover, even if the information we draw on when casting possible futures is 'fit for purpose' then, as human beings, we are not always terribly good at handling it in the complex machine that is cognition.

This book is about how we can combat and avoid some of the pitfalls we are all prone to when handling information in decision making. It was written with a simple aim: to point nurses in the direction of techniques, literature and ideas that (in our experience) are not encountered by nurses during their professional preparation, development or practice. Or, if nurses do come into contact with them (again in our experience) the concepts are not terribly well presented. We have tried to strike a balance between readability, technical detail, practical examples and enough 'science' to satisfy the technocrats. In doing so it is inevitable that some mathematical and scientific notation will be encountered. Some chapters involve some extremely simple calculations. We hope that readers will take the time to engage with these exercises and not to skip over the bits they feel are too statistical or have too many numbers in. Our own research suggests that nurses occasionally avoid more numerate research approaches and decision making aids (in common with the other 98% of the population!). This is a shame, there is much that can be learned from the literature in this area and we sincerely believe that nurses will benefit from being exposed to it.

Finally, a caveat: this book is only an introduction to the academic areas of clinical decision making and judgement. We have striven to show the fundamental basics of techniques, and to do so alongside examples that make them meaningful. The book is categorically *not* a 'how to' manual, nor does it offer the definitive right way to make decisions. Readers will be disappointed if they think that this book will show them how to make 100% 'successful' clinical decisions. Good clinical decisions are born of a consideration of the resources available to you, the wishes of the patient, the cognitive and practical resources you possess by virtue of your clinical expertise and knowledge generated by good quality research. The best decision analysis, clinical guideline, policy capturing mathematical model or decision support software package will only ever fill *some* of the gaps in our decision making armoury. The techniques referred to in this book complement professional judgement and decisions, they are not intended to, and could never, replace such processes.

WHY WORRY ABOUT DECISION MAKING?

A number of policy and professional imperatives mean that nurses have to worry about the decisions they make and the ways in which they make them. In the UK, and the western world generally, there has been an increasing emphasis placed on the need for health care professionals to account for the decisions they make for, with, and on behalf of, their patients. In the UK, several policy initiatives have led to the creation of an evidence based health care culture (Mulhall & Le May, 1999; Box 1.1).

Driving this culture is a societal concern for greater transparency in the decisions taken on its behalf by policy makers and the professionals charged with interpreting and delivering the policies of central

---

Box 1.1 Key milestones in the development of an evidence based NHS culture in the UK

◆ *Working for patients* (Department of Health (DoH), 1989)

◆ *Research for health* (DoH, 1993a)

◆ *Report of the task force on the strategy for research in nursing, midwifery and health visiting* (DoH, 1993b)

◆ *A vision for the future* (DoH, 1993c)

◆ *Supporting research and development in the NHS (the Culyer Report)* (DoH, 1994)

◆ *Methods to promote the implementation of research findings in the NHS* (DoH, 1995)

◆ *Promoting clinical effectiveness* (DoH, 1996a)

◆ *Research and development: Towards an evidence based health service* (DoH, 1996b)

◆ *The new NHS: modern, dependable* (DoH, 1997)

◆ *Towards a strategy for nursing research and development* (DoH, 2000)

All these reports are published by the Department of Health and are available from Her Majesty's Stationery Office, London.

governments. Alongside these rising concerns, society is faced with new and increasingly sophisticated tools with which to acquire the information it perceives it needs. Approximately 25% of the UK population regularly use the Internet, and health service providers are increasingly offering advice and information via these new technologies.

Nurses are taking on new roles: health promoters, giving diagnostic and prognostic information to patients, assessing health risks and screening for early signs of treatable disease. Moreover, in the community many act as public health workers, focusing on whole communities as well as individuals: community profiling, developing health needs assessments, carrying out communicable disease control and undertaking community development work.

These policy drivers have been accompanied by a series of professional drivers, which are shaping the decision making agenda of nurses. The restrictive role based guidance of the old statutory regulatory body of UK nurses has been replaced with guidance on the scope of professional practice (UKCC, 1992). This freedom to practise more autonomously has been accompanied by an increased onus on professional accountability for one's decisions as the cornerstone of a largely self-regulated professional body.

Nursing has also been developing its own internal links between research and professional activity. The relationship between knowledge and decision making has been a crucial element of nursing's attempt to increase its professional status. A number of commentators point to the requirement for professional occupations to possess and develop a relatively esoteric body of knowledge as the basis for practice (Freidson, 1970; Millerson, 1964). How a professional group uses this knowledge determines its position as a profession. MacDonald (1995) suggests that for nursing in particular the interface between nursing's knowledge base and practice (represented by its clinical decisions) is characterised by three constraining factors on nursing attaining 'full' professional status: the nature of nursing knowledge itself, indeterminacy in application and a lack of objectivity in practice.

At the more micro level of individual services and hospitals (in the UK at least) we have seen the evolution of the quality and audit agendas of the 1980s and 1990s into the clinical governance and risk management agendas of the twenty-first century. The Labour government that was elected in 1997 pursued a systematic approach to improving the quality of decisions taken by healthcare professionals in the NHS. The term 'Clinical governance' (DoH, 1998) is intended to encapsulate this approach – officially defined as:

> *'... a framework through which NHS organisations are accountable for continuously improving the quality of their services and safeguarding high standards of care by creating an environment in which excellence in clinical care will flourish'* (DoH, 1998, p. 33).

The Boards of NHS organisations now have a formal duty to ensure that quality is improved and new bodies – the Commission for Health Improvement (CHI) and the National Institute for Clinical Excellence (NICE) – have been established to assist this process (Fig. 1.1).

The UK Department of Health is proposing (for the first time) to examine professional performance and the outcomes of clinical decisions in the NHS and to link this to employment in the NHS. Poor practice, and the decisions that lead to it, will be ever less acceptable. Chief Executives will be accountable for the overall performance of their organisation and they are increasingly likely to scrutinise the quality of provision in individual clinical areas. Evidence based practice and the development of a solid and transparent rationale for decisions will not be an optional extra for doctors, nurses, PAMs (professions allied to medicine) and managers.

In the US, the growth of managed care also has significant implications for professional groups working in health maintenance organisations. As well as challenging the boundaries of clinical freedom and the status of professional judgement, greater supervision of decisions and a fundamental shifting of the professional–patient relationship, managed care

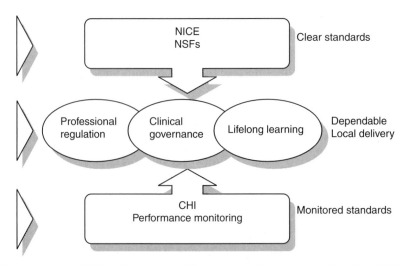

Figure 1.1 The NHS quality structure. Reproduced with permission from DoH (1998).

schemes herald a number of decision challenges for clinicians. The proliferation of clinical guidelines to pre-authorise care delivery, influence management of care and treatment, and guide the management of complex, high-cost cases means that what is no more than a form of decision support has the potential to fundamentally alter the relationship between professional judgement and action. The quality of the guidelines, and the assumptions underpinning them, will have a significant influence on the eventual utility of the end product. As decision analysis and other algorithmic forms of analysing choices often play a part in the guideline development process, then an understanding of how to undertake and apply these techniques will be advantageous to nurses.

WHAT ARE JUDGEMENTS AND DECISIONS?

So what is it about professional nursing practice that makes this book's contribution unique? For us it is the focus on professional choices rather than tasks; knowledge you can use rather than interesting facts about diseases or health (most of which never impact on the management of patients); real life practice rather than the imagined activities of those who see professional status as a good in its own right rather than a means to a desirable end, namely, the higher quality care and treatment of patients. To make this contribution, we should be clear about the parameters of the book and its focus.

In the literature on judgement and decision making, different authors use a number of expressions to describe the same phenomenon. Terms used include, clinical decision making (Field, 1987; Ford et al., 1979; Luker & Kenrick, 1992), clinical judgement (Benner & Tanner, 1987; Itano, 1989), clinical inference (Hammond, 1964), clinical reasoning (Grobe et al., 1991) and diagnostic reasoning (Carnevali et al., 1984; Radwin, 1990). A useful distinction has been made by Dowie (1993, p. 8), who defines judgements as 'the assessment of alternatives' and decisions as 'choosing between alternatives'. In a nursing context, one might make a judgement that a patient's condition has deteriorated and then decide to call a doctor. It is important to recognise that although judgements and decisions can be separated, in health care practice they are interlinked, and therefore often discussed as a single entity.

At this point, it is also worth mentioning that when examining judgement and decision making we can focus on processes and/or outcomes. When considering process, investigators are interested in *how* individuals have reached their judgements and decisions. There is often therefore very little interest in the *outcome* of that process; i.e. how good, bad, accurate or inaccurate it may be. Alternatively, other investigators may be interested in the quality of the outcome of a judgement or decision process, without really considering how that judgement or decision was reached. Again, most research that considers judgement and decision making in nursing and midwifery will have elements of both process and outcome in their studies. In this book, certain chapters focus more on the processes of judgement and decision making (Chs 2, 4 and 6 in particular), whilst others concentrate on the outcomes of that process (Ch. 10, for instance). However, as with most research into judgement and decision making, many of the chapters in the book consider both the process and the outcome of nursing and midwifery judgement and decision making.

THEORIES OF JUDGEMENT AND DECISION MAKING

The study of human judgement and decision making has been the focus of attention for psychologists and others for over half a century. The theories developed from this scrutiny are equally valid for investigating judgement and decision making in nursing and midwifery. The purpose of this section of the chapter is to provide you with a brief overview of some of these theories, together with some of the important concepts that have emerged from them. The remaining chapters in the book build on these theoretical approaches to a greater or lesser extent.

Theories of judgement and decision making can be subdivided into three categories: normative, descriptive and prescriptive. Normative theories assume that an individual is rational and logical, concentrating on how decisions should be made in an ideal world. Usually based on statistical approaches, some of the techniques described in Chapters 5 and 8 in this book have been derived from such normative approaches. Normative theories therefore are often concerned with how 'good' a judgement or a decision is (the outcome) and do not really consider how those judgements or decisions are made in the real world. In contrast, descriptive theories of judgement and decision making try to describe how individuals reach their judgements or decisions. In this way they are more interested in the process of judgement and decision making. Chapter 2 summarises some of the main findings from the large body of work examining how individuals make judgements and decisions. Finally, prescriptive theories try to 'improve' the judgements and decisions of individuals, by examining how individuals actually make judgements and decisions, and trying to help them. Examples of this type of approach are discussed in Chapters 8, 9 and 10.

Information processing

Perhaps the most influential descriptive theory, used as the basis of many of the studies into nursing and midwifery judgement and decision making, is that of information processing (Newell & Simon, 1972). Newell and Simon suggest that human reasoning is 'bounded', in that it is limited by the capacity of the human memory. Subsequent research using information processing theory (also known as the hypothetico-deductive approach) examines how both doctors and nurses reason when making judgements and decisions. This research has suggested that individuals go through a number of phases in their reasoning processes (Elstein et al., 1978; Hamers et al., 1994; Radwin, 1990; Tanner et al., 1987). Box 1.2 outlines the different stages of reasoning when making judgements and decisions, as identified by Elstein et al. (1978), and gives an alternative view of the processes, as identified by Carnevali et al. (1984).

Although there are different numbers of phases in each example in Box 1.2, common features of the reasoning process have been identified in

---

Box 1.2 Stages in the reasoning process

Four stage process (Elstein et al., 1978)

◆ Cue acquisition.
◆ Hypothesis generation.
◆ Cue interpretation.
◆ Hypothesis evaluation.

Seven stage process (Carnevali et al., 1984)

◆ Exposure to pre-encounter data.
◆ Entry to the data search field and shaping the direction of data gathering.
◆ Coalescing of cues into clusters or chunks.
◆ Activating possible diagnostic explanations (hypotheses).
◆ Hypothesis and data directed search of the data field.
◆ Testing diagnostic hypothesis for goodness of fit.
◆ Diagnosis.

a number of studies. With reference to nursing and midwifery, the first stage involves one of gathering preliminary clinical information about the patient (also called the cue acquisition stage). This information can also be gathered before a patient encounter. For instance, you could collect information about the patient's age, medical history, what symptoms they have now (pain, raised temperature, what colour they are, how they move etc.), and what the doctor thinks might be wrong with them.

Following this, you might generate initial and tentative hypotheses (possible explanations for the clinical information you have collected). These are related to the data gathered and cues held in short term memory. From the research that has been carried out, the number of hypotheses generated is normally thought to be between four and six. For instance, you might be looking after a patient who is exhibiting a number of different signs and symptoms (clinical information). You think he might be having a heart attack, although he could just have bad indigestion, or he might just be anxious.

You then move on to the third stage in the reasoning process (interpretation). This involves you interpreting the cues gathered during the data gathering stage and classifying them as confirming, refuting or not contributing to the initial hypotheses (explanations) that you have generated. For instance, some of the clinical information you have collected about your patient – such as a normal ECG – suggests to you that he probably is not having a heart attack even though some of the symptoms he is exhibiting suggest he might be.

Using this classification, the final evaluatory stage involves you weighing up the pros and cons of each possible explanation for your patient's signs and symptoms and choosing the one favoured by the majority of the evidence. Chapter 2 explores in more detail some of the specific ways in which we use information when reasoning to make judgements and decisions, based on this information processing approach.

Intuition and the role of expertise

In the nursing literature in particular, an alternative explanation for how nurses and midwives make judgements and decisions has been equally influential: the idea of intuition. However, just as there is a lack of consensus over the terms used to describe decision making, there is an equal lack of consensus over what is meant by the term intuition. Various definitions of intuition are highlighted in Box 1.3.

Despite the variations in definition, there are commonalties in that intuition is perceived to be a process of reasoning that just 'happens', that

---

Box 1.3 Definitions of intuition

◆ 'Understanding without a rationale' (Benner & Tanner, 1987).

◆ 'A perception of possibilities, meanings and relationships by way of insight' (Gerrity, 1987).

◆ 'Knowledge of a fact or truth, as a whole; immediate possession of knowledge; and knowledge independent of the linear reasoning process' (Rew & Barron, 1987).

◆ 'Immediate knowing of something without the conscious use of reason' (Schrader & Fischer, 1987).

◆ '[A] … process whereby the nurse knows something about a patient that cannot be verbalized, that is verbalized with difficulty or for which the source of knowledge cannot be determined' (Young, 1987).

---

cannot be explained and that is not rational. Perhaps the most well known researcher examining nurse decision making along intuitive lines is Patricia Benner (1984). The main tenet of the intuitive approach is that intuitive judgement distinguishes the expert from the novice; with the expert no longer relying on analytic principles to connect their understanding of the situation to appropriate action. Nursing (as coordinated action) appears intuitive to the outside observer and feels internalised within the practitioner; clinical decisions are the result of an almost unconscious level of cognition (Hamers et al., 1994).

The purpose of this book is to try to provide a pragmatic overview of some of the issues clinical nurses encounter in their everyday practice when making judgements and decisions, and to show how those decisions and judgements might be improved. Despite the undoubted influence of intuitive explanations of judgement and decision making in nursing and midwifery, intuitive theories cannot provide all the answers. This is because, by their nature, intuitive models suggest that knowledge regarding about judgement and decision making is almost impossible to communicate, that it is intangible, and that nurses are unable to express what it is they do. It is therefore difficult to imagine a scenario where nursing's knowledge base becomes a shared resource easily and equally available to all practitioners. Moreover, whilst acknowledging that experts and novices perform differently when making judgements and decisions, it is beyond the scope of this chapter to discuss the issues in detail. The different performance in judgement and decision making tasks of experts is almost certainly connected to their more extensive knowledge base. However, issues around the 'context specific' nature of this knowledge and ability (Crow et al., 1995) limit the ability to generalise and merit a depth of discussion that is beyond this chapter. The Annotated further reading section at the end of this chapter suggests texts with a more in depth discussion of these issues.

The cognitive continuum

A number of commentators highlight that making judgements and decisions is often a combination of stages in the reasoning process (as outlined from the information processing perspective) and intuition. For example, Philips and Rempushki (1985) found that whilst decision making was grounded in the acquisition of data it was far from the linear and monotonic progression assumed by information processing approaches.

An alternative theory or explanation that acknowledges the differences between information processing and intuition is the idea of a cognitive continuum. This theory suggests that reasoning is neither purely intuitive nor purely analytical: that it is located at some point in between. According to the cognitive continuum theory, the major determinants of whether a practitioner utilises a rational or intuitive approach to decision making are primarily determined by the position of the decision task on a continuum. The continuum ranges from pure intuition through system aided judgement to pure analysis (represented by the scientific experiment). A graphical explanation of the continuum can be seen in Figure 1.2. The most appropriate cognitive mode to use for the task in hand depends on three factors: the structure of the task, the number of information cues and the time available to make the judgement or decisions. If a task is poorly structured, with a lot of information cues available and not much time to make the judgement or decision, then intuition is the most appropriate form of cognition to use. If the task is well structured, with few cues and a lot of time available, then a more analytical form of cognition is appropriate. It could be suggested that most healthcare decision making falls somewhere in between these two extremes, and therefore the most appropriate form of cognition for practitioners to use is that of system aided judgements. This type of approach is more 'prescriptive' (helping individuals to improve their judgement and decision making). Chapters 8–10 discuss ways in which this can be facilitated.

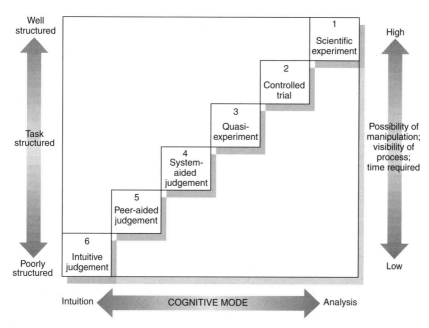

Figure 1.2 The cognitive continuum. Reproduced from Hamm 1988, with permission of Cambridge University Press.

A BRIEF INTRODUCTION TO IMPORTANT CONCEPTS

To understand the whole nature of judgement and decision making in nursing, you need to understand the nature of the concepts that are discussed throughout this book. Box 1.4 lists some of these concepts; it is not an exhaustive list and the definitions offered are 'off the cuff', succinct, versions of terms, expressed in the (workaday) language we use as researchers.

SO WHAT DOES THIS BOOK OFFER? A WALK THROUGH

Chapter 2 highlights those ways in which unaided judgement and decision making can go wrong. The author (Carl Thompson) outlines the short cuts (heuristics) commonly employed by human decision makers and exposes some ways in which the negative effects of using these short cuts can be minimised. The chapter endeavours to outline some of the

Box 1.4 Some words and terms likely to be encountered in later chapters

Action: the behaviour following on from a judgement or decision.

Base rate: sometimes called the prior probability or prevalence. It is usually the true number of patients or subjects in a population who have the disease or characteristic you are interested in. Base rates are usually mentioned in the context of assessing the value of diagnostic tests.

Bias: a tendency to make judgements or decisions on the basis of some pre-formed idea or prejudice.

Bounded rationality: the idea that human beings can never be entirely rational because it is not possible to know in advance exactly what the consequences of choices may be and, even if we could, then humans have only limited computational power.

Clinical information: those characteristics associated with patients and which have a bearing on the diagnosis or management of health and illness. These can be (in the case of non-iatrotropic symptoms) laboratory results, physical manifestations of disease or verbal information provided as part of history taking.

Cognitive continuum: the idea that certain decision tasks merit specific decision making and cognitive styles – ranging from intuition for ill structured, not easily controlled decisions at one end through to the scientific experiment for highly controllable, well structured at the other.

Cognitive processing: the thought processes used when making a judgement or decision.

Cues: see Clinical information, but those features that arise during decision making that have an impact on the eventual decision choice.

Decision: a choice between two alternatives.

Decision rules: the rules or guidelines that an individual uses to guide their decisions (they are internal to the way we think, rather than written down). Often they are not explicit and the individual may not be aware of them.

Decision analysis: a systematic means of charting and considering the risks, benefits, harm and eventualities associated with the various choices comprising a decision task.

Error: a form of decision failure, due either to failure to store or retrieve information for a decision correctly (a slip or a lapse) or some problem at the level of planning or working out a decision (a mistake).

(continued)

Box 1.4 *(continued)*

Evidence: anything you pay attention to when deciding on a course of action. Generally, however, the term refers to knowledge derived from research.

Heuristics: often referred to as 'rules of thumb'. Heuristics are particular strategies that individuals have developed to process a large amount of information efficiently. They 'short cut' having to process a large amount of irrelevant data when making judgements and decisions.

Information processing: a model of cognition based around short term and long term memory. Short term memory houses the stimuli or 'keys' that unlock the factual or experiential information contained in long term memory.

Intuition: immediate knowing of something without the conscious use of reason. It should be noted, though, that the term itself attracts competing definitions.

Judgement: the assessment of alternatives.

Knowledge: the basis of all thought – what we 'know' may come from a variety of different sources, such as formal learning and experience. It has also been suggested that we may have different types of knowledge: the idea of the 'know how' and 'know that'.

Lapse/slip/mistake: see Error.

Probability: chance, or a numerical measure of uncertainty.

Risk: a situation in which there are different possible outcomes, each of which has a known probability of occurring.

Satisficing: in the context of bounded rationality. The term usually refers to the fact that, in real life, decision makers will choose the most feasible option rather than the optimal one as measured by purely rational approaches.

Sensitivity: the ability of a test to identify true positive cases (people who actually have the disease or condition that it is testing for).

Specificity: the ability of a test to identify true negative cases (people who do not have the disease or condition that it is testing for).

Storage: another term for the long term memory. It refers to where we 'keep' our knowledge, such as particular episodes that we have experienced.

Uncertainty: the inability to predict with accuracy what is going to happen. Most judgement and decision making in nursing and midwifery practice is made in conditions of uncertainty – you do not know precisely what the result of your judgement or decision will be.

approaches to errors, slips, lapses and mistakes in decision making and judgement, and present some of the theoretical and empirical justifications for these approaches. It is a largely generic introduction to the idea of error in dealing with clinical uncertainty and draws on a broad body of literature in making its claims that a few simple cognitive 'tips' have the potential to deliver significant benefits in error reduction in practice.

Jane Cioffi's chapter (Ch. 3) takes the theme of exploring judgement further and places it firmly in a nursing context. In fleshing out the picture of judgement painted in Chapter 2, Cioffi manages to illustrate the complex interplay between clinical experience, judgement tasks and accuracy. This chapter also offers some valuable strategic pointers for those nurses keen to explore the limitations and potential of judgement in practice.

The real life judgements of clinicians form the basis of Maxine Offredy's contribution in Chapter 4. Offredy examines the clinical cues, information and features of clinical cases that impact on the judgements of community nurses. As well as highlighting that nurses and doctors use similar processes (and reach similar outcomes) in their diagnostic and treatment clinical decisions, she also manages to show that mapping the complex phenomena of cognition, judgement and decision making calls for a keen methodological imagination. This chapter shows how well constructed scenarios and 'think aloud' techniques are a useful tool in the decision researcher's armoury. Based on her research she provides some hints for promoting the better handling of clinical cues in the diagnosis and treatment planning of common conditions.

The concept of risk in decision theory is central to many people's common sense ideas of the benefits of better handling uncertainty, for example, through risk reduction or more accurate forecasting. In Chapter 5, Dawn Dowding not only develops the concept of risk and rework it for a healthcare audience, but also show how social judgement approaches to decision making under uncertainty can improve the accuracy of the judgements and risk assessments nurses face.

Of course, the best decision support system in the world is rendered useless if targeted at the wrong decisions. The notion that if we are to improve the decisions of nurses then we should have a robust picture of the kinds of decisions that nurses make lies at the heart of Chapter 6. Dorothy McCaughan uses the results of a nursing research study commissioned as part of the UK NHS R&D strategy to illustrate that, far from being some mystical activity open only to nurses, acute care nursing decisions can be captured by a reasonably short typology. Once acknowledged, a wealth of support for decision makers (some generated from nursing research studies but most from other disciplines) becomes available to clinicians. In exploring the decisions of nurses, McCaughan shows that decision makers (and the educators that equip them) need to acquire a range of skills – not all of which are currently widely in evidence in the nursing workforce.

Perhaps the biggest challenge facing nurse decision makers who are aware of the decisions they make, and more importantly the clinical uncertainties that accompany them, is the conversion of these uncertainties into a strategy for action. The technique of developing focused clinical questions forms the start point for Kate Flemming and Mark Fenton's exploration of evidence based approaches to clinical practice and decision making (Ch. 7). As well as addressing the fundamentals of problem identification, searching, critical appraisal and implementation, the two authors offer a simple, example-rich, introduction to some of the statistical terms and quantitative measures used in evidence based approaches to decision making. This section offers a valuable starting point for nurses wanting to add a new dimension to discussions of the benefits, harms, risks and effects of nursing interventions with both colleagues and patients.

Making sense of complex decision problems is not always easy. Even harder is tracking the probabilities associated with decision choices or possible courses of action. Decision analysis offers one means of making such considerations more systematic and is an ideal technique for those nurses facing the kinds of decisions where a choice is not required 'yesterday'. For example, planning a change in service delivery or organisation, or purchasing a new piece of equipment. The technique also has the advantage of improving the decisions made by clinicians in certain situations. Dowding and Thompson (Ch. 8) offer an overview of this valuable approach to systematising judgements and decisions, and provide empirical examples where the approach has worked as well as outlining the pitfalls.

In this era of managed care – in both its explicit US and (more implicit) UK guises – guidelines are becoming an increasing feature of the judgements and decisions of nurses. In Chapter 9, Jo Rycroft-Malone offers the reader an accessible introduction to the nature, development and implications of clinical guidelines. She cuts through much of the terminological confusion in this area to illustrate how to handle guidelines and their development. Moreover, she provides pointers on development, not just where the evidence is strong and the conditions for implementation ideal, but also where professional consensus is the strongest form of evidence available and pragmatism the order of the day.

Robert Crouch gives us a feel for the future of decision support in Chapter 10. The author shows how the power of modern computer technology can make 'real time' decision support a reality for nurses. As well as positing a convincing case for using such technologies, he shows us the myriad of approaches to computerising decision support. The chapter provides a valuable guide through the options available to anyone thinking of utilising new technologies to support the judgements and decisions of clinicians.

All of the chapters have questions for discussion and an annotated further reading included at the end. We would strongly encourage readers to take advantage of the opportunities for discussion, personal or group reflection and knowledge enhancement that these sections offer. If you are a teacher thinking of using the book as part of course work then we would appreciate feedback regarding modifications for future editions.

We hope that the book whets your appetite with regard to this fascinating area. Moreover, we would urge you to seek out the more detailed literature in this area and to find new and imaginative ways of incorporating some of the techniques, skills and tips highlighted in this book in your own practice (and evaluating its impact of course). Finally, it is worth restating that this book is intended only as an introduction. And, whilst not wishing unduly to influence your professional judgement, we sincerely hope that you will make the wise decision to use the book as a starting point for a much longer journey through the literature on improving your clinical decisions and the judgements that feed them.

ANNOTATED FURTHER READING

Dowie, J. & Elstein, A. (1988). *Professional judgement. A reader in clinical decision making.* Cambridge: Cambridge University Press.

An excellent introductory text to all the major debates in decision making and judgement.

Benner, P., Hooper-Kyriakidis, P., & Stannard, D. (1988). *Clinical wisdom and interventions in critical care: A thinking in action approach.* London: WB Saunders.

A nice illustration of expertise in a critical care environment. The book is soundly located in the intuitive-expertise model of decision making and judgement. Whilst rich in descriptive power and normative recommendation, it fails to provide much in the way of a counter position to this stance.

Thompson C. (1999). A conceptual treadmill: The need for 'middle ground' in clinical decision making theory in nursing. *Journal of Advanced Nursing, 30*(5), 1222–1229.

A succinct overview of the major approaches to decision making theory and the rationale for a cognitive continuum.

REFERENCES

Asimov, I (1994). *Asimov's chronology of science and discovery* (updated edition. London: Harper Collins.

Benner, P. (1984). *From novice to expert: excellence and power in clinical nursing practice.* Menlo Park, CA: Addison Wesley.

Benner, P. & Tanner, C.A. (1987). Clinical judgment: How expert nurses use intuition. *American Journal of Nursing, 87*(1), 23–31.

Carnevali, D.L., Mitchell, P.H., Woods, N.F., & Tanner, C.A. (1984). *Diagnostic reasoning in nursing.* Philadelphia: Lippincott.

Crow, R., Chase, J., & Lamond, D. (1995). The cognitive component of nursing assessment: An analysis. *Journal of Advanced Nursing, 22*, 206–212.

Department of Health (1998). *A First Class Service: Quality in the New NHS.* London: HMSO.

Dowie, J. (1993). Clinical decision analysis: Background and introduction. In: Llewelyn, H. & Hopkins, A. (eds), *Analysing how we reach clinical decisions.* London: Royal College of Physicians.

Elstein, A.S., Shulman, L.S., & Sprafka, S.A. (1978). *Medical problem solving: An analysis of clinical reasoning.* Cambridge: Harvard University Press.

Field, P.A. (1987). The impact of nursing theory on the clinical decision making process. *Journal of Advanced Nursing, 12*, 563–571.

Ford, J.A.G., Trygstad-Durland, L.N., & Nelms, B.C. (1979). *Applied decision making for nurses.* St Louis: Mosby.

Freidson, E. (1970). *The profession of medicine.* New York: Dodds Mead.

Gerrity, P. (1987). Perception in nursing: the value of intuition. *Holistic Nursing Practice, 1*(3), 63–71.

Grobe, S.J., Drew, J.A., & Fonteyn, M.E. (1991). A descriptive analysis of experienced nurses' clinical reasoning during a planned task. *Research in Nursing and Health, 14*, 305–314.

Hamers, J.P.H., Abu-Saad H.H., & Halfens R.J.G. (1994). Diagnostic process and decision making in nursing. *Journal of Professional Nursing, 10*(3), 154–163.

Hamm, R.M. (1988). Clinical intuition and clinical analysis: expertise and the cognitive continuum. In: Dowie, J. & Elstein, A. (eds), *Professional judgement: A reader in clinical decision making.* Cambridge: Cambridge University Press, p. 87.

Hammond, K.R. (1964). An approach to the study of clinical inference in nursing: Part II. *Nursing Research, 13*(4), 315–319.

Itano, J.K. (1989). A comparison of the clinical judgment process in experienced registered nurses and student nurses. *Journal of Nursing Education, 28*(3), 120–126.

Luker, K. & Kenrick, M. (1992). An exploratory study of the sources of influence on clinical decisions of community nurses. *Journal of Advanced Nursing, 17*, 457–466.

MacDonald, K.M. (1995). *The sociology of the professions.* London: Sage.

Millerson, G. (1964). *The qualifying association.* London: Routledge and Kegan Paul.

Mulhall, A. & Le May, A. (1999). *Nursing research: Dissemination and implementation.* London: Churchill Livingstone.

Newell, A. & Simon, H.A. (1972). *Human problem solving.* Englewood Cliffs, New Jersey: Prentice Hall.

Philips, L. & Rampushki, V. (1985). A decision making model for diagnosing and intervening in elder abuse and neglect. *Nursing Research, 34*(3), 134–139.

Radwin, L.E. (1990). Research on diagnostic reasoning in nursing. *Nursing Diagnosis, 1*(2), 70–77.

Rew, L. & Barron, E. (1987). Intuition: a neglected hallmark of nursing knowledge. *Advances in Nursing Science, 10*(1), 49–62.

Schrader, B. & Fischer, D. (1987). Using intuitive knowledge in the neonatal intensive care nursery. *Holistic Nursing Practice, 1*(3), 45–51.

Tanner, C.A., Padrick, K.P., Westfall, U.E., & Putzer, D.J. (1987). Diagnostic reasoning strategies of nurses and nursing students. *Nursing Research, 36*(6), 358–363.

UKCC (1992). *The scope of professional practice.* London: UKCC.

Young, C. (1987). Intuition and the nursing process. *Holistic Nursing Practice, 1*(3), 52–62.

2

Human error, bias, decision making and judgement in nursing – the need for a systematic approach

Carl Thompson

KEY ISSUES

◆ Clinical practice involves handling uncertainty in decision making.

◆ The ways in which we make sense of these uncertainties do not always work as we intend.

◆ Errors in decision making can take place at a number of different levels and take different forms.

◆ Decision errors are unavoidable but there are several strategies available to clinicians which can reduce the chances of mistakes, slips and lapses.

THE NATURE OF UNCERTAINTY IN HEALTHCARE DECISION MAKING

Health care is dependent on the clinical decisions of the professionals delivering it. These decisions are often borne of, and accompanied by, uncertainty. To qualify this statement we need to be clear what is meant by uncertainty. Imagine Scenario 2.1.

Scenario 2.1

You are a coronary care staff nurse. A 52-year-old self-employed builder is admitted to your coronary care unit post-myocardial infarction. He recovers well in the initial 2 days post-infarction and you think now would be a good time to start cardiac rehabilitation (in fact, and on reflection, nearly all your patients seem to start the rehabilitation process at this point!). You are aware of the benefits of early rehabilitation and so you broach the subject with the patient and his wife. Whilst telling him what cardiac rehabilitation entails he says, 'Yeah great, but not today – I am too tired, and besides, I have some important decisions to make about my business and I need to be able to concentrate'. You politely, but firmly, suggest that 'perhaps his health is more

(continued)

important ...' (feeling a little miffed that he appears to be spurning your offer of professional support). At this point the man becomes irritated, saying 'OK if it's so good why do we need to start today? What difference will it make if I start in a couple of day's time ... when I want to? I can't believe that watching a video and having a little chat are that important'. It suddenly strikes you that maybe he's right and you do not really know if the 2-day gap is that clinically important after all. You decide to let him cool down and head back to the station ...

Scenario 2.1 contains a number of decisions by the nurse but perhaps the most pertinent is 'deciding to start cardiac rehabilitation on day two post-myocardial infarction'. A number of questions might go through the nurse's mind when making this decision: 'Why do we always seem to start cardiac rehabilitation on day two?', 'Will it matter if the patient doesn't get rehab on this day?', 'Am I explaining the benefits of rehabilitation in the best way?'. It is these clinical questions that are the crux of uncertainty in clinical decision making: the outcomes or consequences of your decision making cannot ever be predicted with complete certainty in health care.

McCaughan (Ch. 6) shows how such uncertainty is present in the kinds of decisions acute care nurses commonly face. Flemming and Fenton (Ch. 7) show how such uncertainties can be reduced by developing evidence based focused clinical questions. What both these chapters illustrate is that uncertainty differs according to the nature of the decisions faced. For example:

◆ *Planning* a patient's care involves assessing the *likelihood* of a challenge to their health status (e.g. 'If I stop this person's intravenous infusion, how likely are they to become dehydrated?').
◆ In this era of nurse consultants and nurse prescribing, you might make a medical *diagnosis* such as psoriasis or asthma (e.g. 'How likely is it that this person's symptoms are being caused by psoriasis or asthma?').
◆ In selecting *interventions* to meet needs or help treat a disease you will want to know the *probability* that one of the decision choices is likely to deliver the outcome you and the patient actually want (e.g. 'If I choose this wound dressing how likely is it that the pressure sore will heal?').

◆ You will wish to know the *chances* of bad outcomes if you watchfully wait (e.g. 'If I don't do anything now how likely is it that this person will get worse?').

In trying to reduce these kinds of uncertainties you may use a number of information seeking strategies:

◆ You will almost certainly draw on your previous experience. But you might be able to generalise from only two or three other patients like this you have seen.
◆ You might ask colleagues whose advice you trust. However, you do not know where they are getting their information from and it could be that their experience is no more extensive than yours.
◆ You might decide to 'look at the literature'. However, textbooks on your unit are already out of date (on average by around 10–15 years). You also need some idea of the right kind of research evidence to consult for the kind of decision you face, together with some way of condensing the results and a way of factoring in your patient's preferences. It is therefore unlikely that the literature available to you will help you much.

Each of these strategies will deliver information that will appear to reduce the uncertainties you face by providing you with some detail about how likely the different outcomes are to occur. However, as we shall see, there are problems in the ways that human beings process the information provided by such sources. Also, most of the strategies healthcare professionals employ to help reduce clinical uncertainty do not necessarily help prevent errors in decision making itself.

THE NATURE OF ERROR IN HEALTHCARE DECISION MAKING

Before the chapter progresses any further, a quick task. Try and work out the answer to the sum below, do not use a calculator and take only 3 seconds:

$$1 \times 2 \times 3 \times 4 \times 5 \times 6 \times 7 \times 8 =$$

We will see later in the chapter why this sum is relevant.

When we make decisions we choose between discrete options or actions. The choices made are intentional – by making a decision we are acting on a prior intention. It is not possible to make an error without this

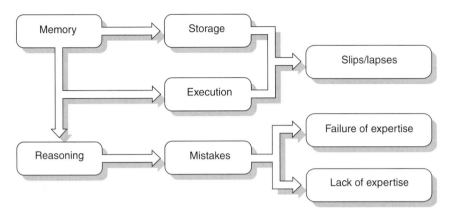

Figure 2.1 A summary of error types.

prior intention in place. Reason (1998, p. 9) defines error as 'a generic term encompassing all those occasions in which a planned sequence of mental or physical activities fails to achieve its intended outcome, and when these failures cannot be attributed to the intervention of some chance agency'.

Errors (or decision failures) can occur at a number of levels (Fig. 2.1). Slips or lapses have been defined as 'errors which result from some failures in the execution and/or storage stage of an action sequence, regardless of whether or not the plan which guided them was adequate to achieve its objective' (Reason, 1998). They occur if the actions associated with a decision do not proceed as planned (for example, you forget to consent the patient despite going to the bedside to do so).

Mistakes have been defined as 'deficiencies or failures in the judgmental and/or inferential processes involved in the selection of an objective or in the specification of the means to achieve it, irrespective of whether or not the actions directed by this decision-scheme run according to plan' (Reason, 1998). They occur when your thinking about a decision is faulty (for example, you think that a patient's chest pain is a symptom of indigestion and fail to realise he is actually having a heart attack). Of course, if intended actions proceed as you wish, and achieve the desired ends, then this is a successful decision and there is no problem.

Mistakes can be further subdivided into:

◆ *Failures of expertise* – nurses bring a pre-established plan or solution to a decision based on their expertise in the area, but do so inappropriately.
◆ *Failures due to a lack of expertise* – nurses have no pre-formed plan (perhaps because they have never encountered this kind of

patient before), and have to develop a solution or plan from first principles or whatever knowledge is available and perceived as relevant.

TOWARDS A FRAMEWORK FOR DECISION MAKING AND ERROR PREVENTION

I am sure readers will recognise instances in their own practice where slips, lapses and mistakes have occurred. At this point, however, we need to step back and remember that this book is about 'real life' decision making. There are four characteristics of human beings and their decision making that prevent wholesale acceptance of this simple model.

Firstly, slips, lapses and mistakes operate at different levels of thinking. Slips and lapses occur at the level of unintended actions often in the form of 'taking your eye off the ball' or (in the language of behavioural decision theorists) 'deficient attentional monitoring'. Mistakes, on the other hand, involve processing information and planning goal achievement mechanisms (i.e. they involve problems with how you use or process information when you are making judgements and decisions). Given this difference, mistakes should be more advanced than errors, more complex and possibly more serious. However, this is not always the case; slips and lapses can also be what has been termed 'strong but wrong' (Reason, 1998, p. 54) and based more on previous practice than the circumstances of the current decision situation. For example, nurses who are used to an older defibrillation device and who consistently administer low voltage shocks in a cardiac arrest because they failed to recognise the difference in the location of the voltage selectors between the old and new devices.

Secondly, the distinctions between slips, lapses and mistakes are often not as clearly defined as one would expect. For example, consider the (real) health care incidents in Scenarios 2.2 and 2.3.

Scenario 2.2

A junior staff nurse working in a busy coronary care unit was handed a syringe by a doctor and asked to give the morphine to 'that patient'. The nurse went to the patient and gave the morphine as instructed. A little time later the doctor said to the nurse 'But that patient is still in pain'. At which point the nurse realised that the morphine had been given to the wrong patient.

Scenario 2.3

A paediatric resuscitation team is attempting to revive a 1-year-old baby. The doctor calls for calcium chloride and the nurse passes potassium chloride. The baby subsequently dies.

These scenarios illustrate that errors are complex multidimensional entities where mistakes, slips and lapses can all occur in the same incident. They also highlight the possibility that relatively simple techniques (such as reciting back instructions for clarification when drug doses have been ordered) can help.

Thirdly, human beings are inveterate 'pattern matchers' (Deutsch et al., 1994) with an in built capacity to override rational solutions via a series of cognitive shortcuts or heuristics (more on this later).

Fourthly, we know that decisions are necessarily satisfied (as highlighted in Ch. 1) because information is nearly always incomplete and rationality 'bounded' (Simon, 1982).

Having acknowledged these limitations in the model we can now rework our view of error and suggest that lapses and slips take place at the level of skills (and the application of those skills to patients; Box 2.1), whilst mistakes can operate on two levels: decision rules and the handling of knowledge (Boxes 2.2 and 2.3).

Reason (1998) links this conceptual split to a three level 'generic' model of decision making (Fig. 2.2) and, in doing so, opens up the possibility of solutions to some of the common error types.

Skills based failure

Inattention based failures are due to a lack of attention at crucial moments in clinical practice (e.g. not paying attention when giving an intravenous

---

Box 2.1 Skills based performance

◆ Inattention.
◆ Double capture.
◆ Omission following interruption.
◆ Reduced intentionality.
◆ Perceptual confusion.
◆ Interference errors.

Box 2.2 Rule based performance

- ◆ Misapplication of good decision rules.
- ◆ First exceptions.
- ◆ Countersigns and non-signs.
- ◆ Informational overload.
- ◆ Rule strength.
- ◆ General rules.
- ◆ Redundancy.
- ◆ Rigidity.
- ◆ Application of bad rules.
- ◆ Encoding deficiencies.
- ◆ Action deficiencies.

Box 2.3 Knowledge based performance

- ◆ Over confidence.
- ◆ Hindsight bias.
- ◆ Base rate neglect.
- ◆ Availability heuristic.
- ◆ Anchoring bias.

---

drug, so you haven't realised that the drug is going into the patient's tissues).

Double capture failures occur when people focus on some event that distracts or preoccupies in a decision situation (e.g. being so preoccupied by a patient's cardiac monitor that you fail to realise that he's removed his oxygen and his saturation levels are dropping).

Interruptions can be problematic and lead to slips and lapses (e.g. 'I was recalculating the drug dose because I wasn't sure it was right, then the station phone rang, I answered it, and then gave the original [wrong] dose').

Failure due to reduced intentionality happens when there is a gap between intending to do something and carrying it out (e.g. 'I knew that I wanted to tell the patient about cardiac rehabilitation but when I got in there his relatives were there and I started asking about his social support

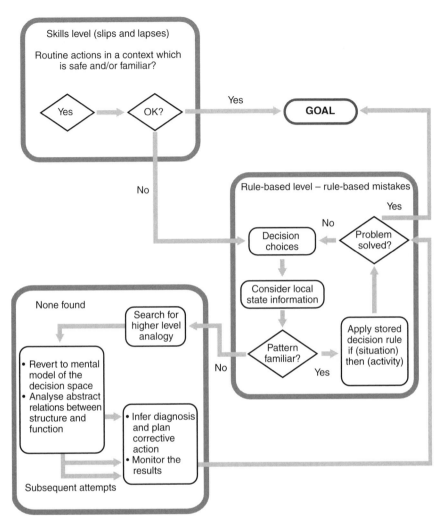

Figure 2.2 A generic decision error system. Reason (1988).

networks instead'). In their lapse form these kinds of errors commonly take the form of 'I know I should be doing something but can't remember what'.

Perceptual confusion occurs when the 'matching' of action to routinely recognised situations gets confused. This tends to occur when cue recognition (the information you focus on to inform your decision) becomes so automatic that rough approximations suffice (e.g. 'I meant to get the water ampoule but grabbed sodium chloride instead … they look so similar').

Interference errors occur when attempting multiple tasks and mixing up action sequences (e.g. 'I was desperate to finish the drugs and this patient kept going on about wanting the toilet and so I put his pills in the toilet').

Rule based failure

When people try and make sense of situations and decide what to do (especially in familiar situations) they often apply a series of decision rules. Commonly these are in the form of, 'if … a situation matches X … then … it merits action Y'. Often, people have many rules that could apply. How and if they decide to apply them depends on a number of factors:

◆ the rule has to match a salient feature of the decision environment
◆ the strength of the rule (for example, how often it has proved successful in the past)
◆ the degree of specificity associated with the decision, i.e. the amount of approximation associated with deciding if the rule 'fits'
◆ the amount of support that the rule receives from other – competing – decision rules.

The upshot of these characteristics is that decision rules exist on a continuum ranging from good (i.e. they match, they are strong, they are specific and they attract support) through to bad (they do not). The failure of decision rules can be traced to two effects: the misapplication of good rules, or the application of bad rules.

Misapplying good rules

Because one of the characteristics of choosing to deploy a good decision rule is its utility (derived from success in past experiences), then the first time an individual encounters an exception to a general rule they are prone to employ a strong, but still wrong, decision rule. For example, imagine that cardiac monitors on a CCU are routinely set to alarm at a tachycardia of more than 100 bpm, and nurses commonly react automatically, by glancing at the reading (for signs of a life threatening arrhythmia). Then, having established that they haven't got one (semi-automatically) the nurses reset the alarm. It is quite possible to imagine that the first time the nurses encounter an alarm where the sinus tachycardia is more than 160 bpm they might still react the same way – at least initially. They have learned (the general decision rule) that the alarm is associated with a non-threatening sinus tachycardia and so can safely be reset.

Obviously, they will (indeed, should) adjust their decision rule after this first exception – as long as they recognise the error.

Whether we employ a particular decision rule depends on the degree of fit between the rules and the decision situation faced. Where there is noise in the decision situation, or where competing (irrelevant) information cues impact on our ability to establish this fit, then the wrong rules can be brought into play. This noise is compounded by the volume of information presented in real life decision making. For example, consider the decision of whether a patient in your care needs medical rather than nursing attention. The information cues one might need are physical observations such as temperature, pulse, respiration and blood pressure; an intuitive gut feeling (most likely to derive from experience with other patients); advice from colleagues; information provided by the patient; and the formal/informal protocols in the unit. These cues are all potentially contradictory and can (if unfiltered) lead to confused decision making.

Rules with a proven track record of success will necessarily be given a higher weighting in decisions. Reason (1998) uses the analogy of a horse race: the rule with the best form has the highest chance of winning future races. However, sometimes these 'superstrong' rules are applied without regard to the other factors determining utility such as the degree of 'fit', or support from other decision rules. It is possible to see how other decision rules can be seen as good for lots of situations, i.e. they are general rules, whilst others are more specific. People are often attracted to the application of general decision rules rather than specific ones. For example, neonatal nurses administered high concentration oxygen to preterm babies for many years in the belief that oxygen is good for humans (usually a fairly reliable decision rule). However, the correct and specific decision rule for that situation should have been that high concentration oxygen for neonates is bad because it makes them blind. Despite the experiences of watching babies acquire blindness, the decision rule held for some years.

Humans learn to break down complex decision or problem situations into manageable chunks. In the long run we recognise that only key bits of information are genuinely useful in reducing uncertainty. The converse situation is that we recognise that the information attached to decision situations can often be redundant. This learning process encourages people to focus rigidly on those bits of information that have worked in the past but that might not be the most pertinent for the specific situation faced (i.e. humans match patterns of information to help them make a decision). It takes time and effort for individuals to reject 'going with what they know', even in the face of new, better or more elegant decision rules: they are cognitively conservative (Hammond, 1964).

Applying bad rules

Decision failures based on the application of bad rules to a situation can be traced to two kinds of flaws: encoding and action. Encoding means making sense of complex situations (i.e. putting them into a format we can use in practical decision making). Encoding failures take a number of forms but three common problems are at their core.

First, when developing skills, human beings have difficulty managing two or more tasks simultaneously. For example, take the task of, and decisions involved in, driving a car. In the early stages of your driving career, navigating a safe path on the road and maintaining speed appear almost mutually exclusive. Humans concentrate on just one aspect of the skill and place the others on one side in order to keep the task manageable. As your skills develop you are able to pay more attention to the aspect placed on one side and eventually you are able to do both automatically. For a clinical example, consider the process of your first intramuscular injection and the decision processes that got placed on one side of the cognitive workspace whilst learning to do it all 'seamlessly': '... Select the right upper quadrant of the right buttock ... hands in the wrong place ... oops! Have to move the hand to be able to operate the plunger ... if I let go of the syringe will it fall out?... there's a bit of blood in the barrel ...' and so on.

It is likely that many students are able to give accurate intramuscular injections but that other elements of the total injection experience are given a lower weighting – speed, for example. In relation to encoding problems this means that individuals may focus on only one aspect of the task, rather than the whole thing.

Humans also seem to have problems judging concepts. We deploy a kind of 'intuitive' reasoning that is often erroneous. This is particularly true of the physical world and, as nursing depends in part on observing the physical world (for example, looking at a patient's colour or listening to heart or chest sounds), then this flaw is pertinent. Reason (1998) points to the example of college students who watched a ball being fired from a coiled tube. They reasoned (intuitively) that the trajectory of the ball coming out was curved (as the tube was coiled), which is a wrong choice. The use of intuitive decision choices in the physical world can often lead to wrong decisions.

Many general rules are often protected by domain specific exception rules (i.e. rules that apply in all situations apart from X). Reason (1998) gives the example of the social preservation of negative stereotypes as an instance where the exception serves to protect the bad general rule: 'some of my best friends are ...'. Here the fact that the individual knows one or two people who 'fit' their view of the stereotype (even if the vast majority of people do not) proves to the individual that the stereotype has some utility. Clearly this is a bad rule for professionals to employ.

Decision rules usually involve action that can vary from simply wrong to inadvisable. Applying home made strategies for calculating drips per minute in intravenous fluid giving sets (the 'I just know when it's right' approach) would be a wrong action component in a decision rule. At the middle level, the use of false economies is often a major cause of bad decision rules. For example, reusing disposable gloves on different patients to save money will have potentially serious implications, with the harm eventually outweighing the economic benefits. At the level of the inadvisable, the belief that driving too close to the car in front is an effective means of getting the person to pull over and for you to get to a meeting sooner is clearly a bad decision rule. It may sometimes work and reinforce the rule but in the long run is inadvisable and will eventually lead to a collision.

Failure at the knowledge based level: heuristics and biases

This chapter is en route to providing some practical tips to combating failure in decision making. Most professional practice involves the application of knowledge to a problem. This is a positive thing in that knowledge of the right sort (e.g. research) brings with it potentially better outcomes for the patient. However, in processing and applying the knowledge we use in practice we are prone to a different set of failures to the ones highlighted thus far.

Over confidence

Individuals are often over confident when assessing the correctness of their knowledge. Ironically, this often occurs in situations when we have least knowledge. Clearly this is problematic in relation to nurses' clinical decision making, as decision making is the time when uncertainty (and an associated lack of confidence) is most likely to arise. There are a number of classic laboratory studies showing that individuals are over confident in a variety of cognitive settings. These include two-choice general knowledge questions (Gigerenzer, 1991; Lichenstein & Fischoff, 1977); impossible tasks involving perception, such as assigning the continents of authors by their handwriting or predicting the rise of stocks based on

---

Box 2.4 Ten questions for examining confidence

1. What is a healthy blood clotting time (in seconds) for an adult?
2. What is a normal chloride figure in blood plasma?
3. What is a normal pH for blood?
4. What is the specific gravity of urine?
5. How many calories do 100 g of carbohydrate provide?
6. What are the chances of an asymptomatic individual from a non-caucasian ethnic group having organic coronary artery disease?
7. In what year did Florence Nightingale return from the Crimea?
8. What is the number of visits made by district nurses in a day in the NHS?
9. Iceland legalised abortion in which year?
10. What percentage of individuals with herpes simplex virus (type 1) are asymptomatic?

---

limited knowledge of previous performance (Fischoff, 1975; Lichenstein & Fischoff, 1977) and guessing the true value of a quantity (Lichenstein & Fischoff, 1977). However, nurses commonly do not work in the controlled environment of the psychology laboratory and so how might this kind of over confidence manifest itself? We can demonstrate the over confidence heuristic quite easily.

There are ten questions in Box 2.4. Look at these questions and then write down the range in which you can be 90% sure that the answer lies. For example 'What proportion of patients are successfully resuscitated on television hospital dramas?'. I am 90% sure I think that the bottom figure is 85% and the top is 99%, so the answer lies between 85% and 99%. If the true answer is 65% then I was wrong on this occasion (in fact, I do not know what the true answer is, this is only an example!). At the 90% level you should get nine of the ten questions correct. Try not to be under confident by putting your top and bottom estimates too far apart – you would not be able to do this in real life practice (imagine saying 'Your chances of a recovery are between 5% and 95% Mrs Smith'). The answers to the questions are on page 43.

How did you do? 5, 6, 7, 8 out of 10? Or less? Hopefully this demonstrated that even in an area of knowledge (health care) in which we have a modicum of expertise, over confidence is common. Later in the chapter we will see how you can combat this tendency.

Hindsight bias

Most nurses at some point will be aware of exhortations to be more 'reflective'. Our experiences amount to rich repositories of information that can be used in our clinical decisions. Research conducted by the University of York has demonstrated that nurses' primary source of evidence for practice is their own experience and that of their colleagues. Using experience in this way can be a necessary and positive force in decision making. However, experience alone is not a sufficient prerequisite for good clinical decisions. Again, in the laboratory it has been shown that hindsight artificially increases the estimate of the outcomes of events that happened in the past (Fischoff, 1975), increases the estimated chances of medical diagnoses (Arkes et al., 1966) and produces favourable distortions of memory. Jones (1995) has suggested that nurses are also prone to hindsight bias, with knowledge of a patient's medical diagnosis affecting their judgement. Poulton (1994) uses the example of historians to illustrate that knowing the outcome of events makes it impossible to be fair when reflecting on the causes of those events: people will search for detailed causal connections, selectively recall key events and reconstruct scenarios that are different to those constructed when the outcome was unknown. A clinical parallel can be found here, in the use of clinical supervision as a device for improving the quality of decisions made by practitioners. If the supervision session takes place according to a framework that is naïve and unsophisticated (i.e. doesn't try and counter hindsight bias) then it is likely that the power of the technique will be limited. Again we will encounter some specific advice on how to counter this tendency later in the chapter.

Base rate neglect

Healthcare professionals have a tendency to neglect the underlying base rates of disease or symptoms when diagnosing or treating illnesses (Dowie & Elstein, 1988). The classic example was illustrated by Kahneman and Tversky (1973), who examined the biases of people when presented with stereotypical descriptions of individuals. In their experiment they presented people with the knowledge that there was a 30 : 70 ratio of engineers to lawyers in a sample. From these figures you can see that there is a smaller statistical probability that any one individual (if selected) will be an engineer. However, they then presented subjects with descriptions of individuals that matched stereotypes of engineers: 'Jack is a 45-year-old man, married with four children, conservative, careful and ambitious. Not interested in political or social issues and spends his hobby time doing carpentry and mathematical puzzles'. Most people stated that the person was likely to be one of the (much smaller) group of 30 engineers. Of course, this information represents our own biases based on qualitative information. The subjects would have been better off arguing that the individual is a lawyer because he has a higher chance of being in that group (2.3 to 1).

Base rates are important from a clinical perspective. For instance, imagine a situation in which a test for particular disease (and ordering tests will become a formal part of the nurse's role in the 'new NHS') has a very high false positive rate (the test is positive but the person does not have the disease) and yet the actual condition or the base rate of the disease in the population as a whole is very low. What this means is that most people testing positive do not really have the disease or condition – the test is not all that useful. If you ignore the base rates in a population you run the risk of misinterpreting the real chances of having a disease or the significance of the signs observed (this is also discussed in Ch. 5).

There is some evidence (albeit methodologically limited) that nurses and doctors do manage to pay attention to base rates. Cioffi (1997) cites the work of Benner and Tanner (1987) as symptomatic of nurses' recognition that base rates impact on decisions. Certainly, my own team's work with nurses suggests that comparisons to other patients' symptom or condition rates such as, 'nine out of ten patients will have a mildly raised blood sugar post-MI' are common in many nurses' reasoning processes. The problem here is that whilst experience encourages attention to base rates (Christensen-Szalanski, 1981) it is limited as a knowledge source. Amassing enough experience with similar patients is problematic enough but, as we have seen, the role of hindsight and other forms of bias mean that such experience is likely to be distorted by knowledge of the patient in front of you. There are strategies one can utilise though, which, when combined with quality research information (see Ch. 7) to 'help fill in the cognitive gaps', can provide aids to reaching decisions.

Availability heuristics

People tend to use information that is closest to hand when making decisions (Friedlander & Stockman, 1983). The problem with this approach is that what is closest to hand is not necessarily the same for each individual and so variation in decisions can result. Again this is easily demonstrated:

◆ Find a blank piece of paper and a pen.
◆ Now, examine the 20 words in Box 2.5 one at a time. Look at them only once – do not re-read them and do not go over the list again.
◆ Cover up the list.

Box 2.5

Flange

Routemaster

Laggard

Sausages

Automaton

Approach

Antichrist

Research

Slipper

Haggle

Fridge

Locomotive

Bracket

Confused

Telesales

Professor

Stool pigeon

Hale

Banquet

Irrelevance

◆ Without looking at Box 2.5, write as many of the words as you can remember on the blank sheet of paper.

◆ When you have finished, draw the blank graph in Figure 2.3 on your sheet of paper.

◆ Now, how many of the first four words did you remember? Divide this figure by 20 and mark it on the graph over the 1 to 4 label on the X axis.

◆ How many of next four did you get right? Again, divide this figure by 20 and plot it over the 5 to 8 label on the X axis. Do this another three times until each label has a mark (the probability that you will recall this word) over it.

◆ Now draw a line from each mark down to the X axis on the graph to graphically represent the probability of recall for that group of words.

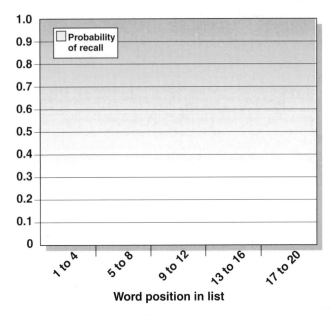

Figure 2.3 Blank graph for the availability heuristic.

What you should see is higher lines (or bars) at one or other end of the X axis. This shows that you are more likely to recall information from the beginning of the list (the primacy effect) or from the end of the list (the recency effect). This is common, and demonstrates that people recall information differently. Try doing this with a friend or colleague and see if they have different results. This means that you are more likely to recall recent similar instances of a decision problem to that in front of you, which may not necessarily be the most appropriate match for this particular problem.

Anchoring bias

When people make decisions they draw on anchors to help them. Anchors are cognitive reference points from which people work outwards. Cioffi (1997) uses the example of the midwife who describes the colour of a baby following an assessment for jaundice 'every baby has a colour of his own ... hopefully every baby is pink, or if they're a couple of days old, they may be a little yellow'. For this nurse, the initial anchors are her colour values of 'pink' and 'yellow', from which she can work outwards to describe the jaundice. Cioffi implies that this kind of heuristic is valuable, even desirable, in professional practice. Certainly, there is little doubt that some approaches to professional expertise (the Dreyfus's (1986) and Benner

(1984) models) imply that these anchors are legitimate and useful. Experts are commonly classified as experts because they are skilled in deploying these anchors (often as a result of considerable clinical experience).

However, not all anchoring heuristics are desirable. For example, try the following calculation, do not use a calculator, do not look down the page and only take three seconds:

$$8 \times 7 \times 6 \times 5 \times 4 \times 3 \times 2 \times 1 =$$

Did you arrive at a larger figure than for the sum presented earlier (page 24)? If you did (and do not worry if you did not) it is because people tend towards smaller anchors in numerical problems that start with small numbers; the converse is true for problems with large starting numbers (Tversky & Kahneman, 1973). As long as the anchors are of good quality and reliable then this heuristic can be a useful part of the professional cognitive toolkit. The problem with such anchors, as we have seen, is that other kinds of heuristic and error types can distort their construction and it is difficult to amass enough experiences of a similar nature to construct them for every situation. The correct answer for the sum, by the way, is 40 320.

COMBATING BIAS AND ERROR: WHAT CAN BE DONE?

There are a number of relatively simple tips that one can employ as a clinician to try and combat these tendencies towards bias in human reasoning and so reduce the chances of error. Some of these tips are presented in the excellent Nottingham University Behavioural Sciences teaching package on clinical decision making (see http://www.ccc.nottingham.ac.uk/~mczwww/tltp/decis.htm).

At the level of skills based error, good environmental management can help to reduce the number of slips and lapses. For instance, reducing interruptions from external sources, trying not to have frequent changes of activity and not rushing through (and into) tasks without first quickly reflecting on the importance of each to the patient or yourself.

You can try to minimise the chances of slips, lapses and mistakes by employing decision rules that have been validated and will benefit the vast majority of patients. National evidence based clinical guidelines (e.g. the Royal College of Nursing's leg ulcer guidelines) (RCN 1988) are good examples of these. Locally, decision support tools such as evidence based protocols might provide the best source of decision support in times of uncertainty. Of course, such technologies should be appraised critically to ascertain the quality of production, implications of use, and the applicability to the patient in front of you (see Chs 7and 9). Individual decision rules can be challenged successfully via reflective techniques conducted 'on the hoof', referred to as 'reflection in action' by Benner et al. (1999). Questioning our assumptions about patients at the time of a decision can be useful; as can imagining the 'long run' consequences of a decision choice (i.e. what would happen if you took the same decision for other similar patients over time).

As professionals who apply knowledge, the most significant challenge to reducing practice based errors can be at the level of knowledge based failure. Heuristics are simultaneously an aid to reducing uncertainty and also the main cause of bias and poor decisions. So how can we work with them? One way of harnessing the normative rules associated with heuristics and reducing the bias associated with the 'real life' approaches adopted by humans is to use formal decision aids. Decision analysis (see Ch. 8), decision support software (Ch. 10) and expert referral can all help for some decisions but they can be time consuming, involve excessive commitment of resources and be difficult to use at first. Thankfully there are some prosaic yet powerful techniques that can be utilised at the individual level of applying one's professional knowledge:

◆ give due weight to base rates
◆ combat over confidence and availability
◆ combat other knowledge use biases.

Giving due weight to base rates

In the absence of quality diagnostic tests (of which there are few in nursing), base rates can be the best indication of a particular disease or condition. Consider Scenario 2.4.

Scenario 2.4

You take a urine sample from a patient and it shows raised sugar levels. You know from experience that only about 1 in 100 such cases are actually indicative of diabetes (Table 2.1). To be sure though, you decide to persuade the ward team to use the more accurate fasting blood sugar test. This test correctly identifies 80% of diabetics and 90% of non-diabetics. So what are the chances of the patient having diabetes?

| 100% | 90% | 80% | 72% | 7.5% | 1% |

Fasting blood sugar results	True diabetic status		Population
	Diabetic	**Non-diabetic**	
Diabetic	0.8	9.9	10.7
Non-diabetic	0.2	89.1	89.3
Population	1	99	100

Table 2.1 Taking accounts of base rates: Bayes' theorem

The answer is 7.5%. Did you get it right? If you did, do you know why? If you answered 80% or 72%, you probably made the common mistake of confusing the chances of having a positive test result given the patient has diabetes (which is how most researchers present results) with the chances of having diabetes given a positive test result (which is how most nurses need information for decision making). If you think about it, you know that only around 1% of urine tests are indicative of diabetes (your experience tells you this). What the fasting blood sugar test is picking up is 80% (see Table 2.1) of these (for more discussion of this issue, see the more detailed treatment of sensitivity and specificity in Ch. 5).

Critical appraisal of tests that you order can also be really useful. By looking at the evidence for a test you can ascertain whether the test was developed and tested in settings that make it unsuitable for your uses. For example, if fasting blood sugar is tested in a setting in which nearly 100% of patients are diabetic (say a diabetes ward), then it is unlikely to be much use as a device for identifying diabetics in the community.

Combating over confidence and availability

'Reflection in action' is probably not an adequate mechanism for avoiding errors by itself but, by questioning whether you really are 90% sure, or if it is more like 75%, then you can revise your estimates of correctness. This technique also helps you decide whether you really know the answer or if further evidence gathering is necessary. When questioning your level of confidence (and revising as necessary) you should also make the effort to combat the effects of primacy and recency. So be aware that the information that jumps straight to the front of your mind when trying to grapple with the uncertainties in a clinical decision may not necessarily be the best evidence – actively question the information and try and think of alternatives.

Combating other knowledge use biases

The best strategy is to question your instincts. The impact of hindsight bias (once you know the outcome of previous cases assigning the wrong causal probabilities and constructing the wrong scenarios) can be down-played by asking the question 'What might have happened if another outcome had occurred in this case?'.

Anchoring heuristics should be challenged by recognising that just because something sounds plausible, or fits a stereotype, it is not neces-sarily more likely to happen. Nursing has a culture of individualised care but most nurses can think of examples of stereotypes determining the approach to a patient's management. For example 'the "wimp" in bed four who is taking too long to get out of bed post-hernia repair' or 'the unemployed father whose daughter's broken arm was "probably" a non-accidental injury' (both of these examples are drawn from my own experi-ences in practice). It is probability that indicates the chances of things happening rather than qualitative indicators of bias. Stereotypical views of patients are one of the most unacceptable faces of healthcare delivery and a major block on quality decision making.

By framing decisions in different ways we can reach different conclu-sions. For example, it is quite likely that the nurse involved in Scenario 2.1 (page 22) had the relative benefits of cardiac rehabilitation at the front of her mind when asking the patient to participate. However, given his response, it may be just as feasible that the patient was more concerned with the absolute risks associated with not partaking (see Ch. 7 for a dis-cussion of absolute and relative risk and benefits). With some slippage in both party's positions and some creative (evidence based) communication from the nurse, the situation may have been different.

CONCLUSION

This chapter has demonstrated that, when making decisions, nurses (like all humans) are subject to uncertainty, error and heuristic short cuts. Unfortunately, it has also shown that these heuristics (or short cuts) are not infallible and can actually introduce unhelpful biases into our decision making. This is problematic, as errors in health care are becoming increasingly visible and rising public expectation demands that profes-sionals learn from mistakes and take corrective action. Many of the tech-niques in this book, such as decision analysis, evidence based decision making and computerised decision support, are designed to combat the tendencies of human decision makers and, as such, are valuable. However, not all decisions are amenable to the potential benefits these technologies offer. Probably most 'real life' nursing and midwifery decisions require readily accessible techniques that can be applied at the bedside, ward or treatment room. This chapter has highlighted just a few of the simple techniques nurses can utilise to reduce bias and error, together with some common pitfalls to be aware of and avoid if possible. Most of these skills can be picked up quickly, discussed with colleagues, and, with practice, mastered and embedded in clinical practice decisions. None of the techniques constitute 'rocket science' and even the most advanced require no more than simple mathematical skills.

This chapter is only a starting point and readers are advised to consult the excellent, but more detailed, texts in the list of annotated further reading if they are serious about acquiring the knowledge and skills to really develop their professional decision making.

ANSWERS TO THE QUESTIONS IN BOX 2.4

1. Anywhere in the range 240–600 s

2. Anywhere in the range 95–105 mmol/l

3. Anywhere in the range 7.35–7.45

4. Anywhere in the range 1002–1040°

5. 400

6. 3.2%

7. 1856

8. 100 000

9. 1935

10. 60%

Sources for the answers

Dingwall, R., Rafferty, A.M., & Webster, C. (1988). *Introduction to the social history of nursing*. London: Routledge.
Kasner, K. & Tindall, D. (1984). *Nurses dictionary*. London: Bailliere Tindall.
New England Journal of Medicine (1999). *341*, 1432–1438.
Silagy, C. & Haines, A. (1998). *Evidence based primary care*. London: BMJ Publishing.

QUESTIONS FOR DISCUSSION

◆ Reflect on a healthcare decision you took in the past that did not turn out as you expected. Could you have handled things differently? How might some of the strategies presented here have helped?

◆ Look at some prevalence audit data for common conditions on your ward, unit or community 'patch' (diabetes, heart disease or asthma perhaps). Having established some base rates for these conditions on your unit or area, why not look at how useful (sensitive and specific) some of the common diagnostic tests you use are (routine urinalysis perhaps). How useful are they *really*?

◆ How can you change the ways you work in order to reduce your chances of making errors? Can you think of a way of adapting your clinical audit or clinical governance agenda to try and monitor progress?

ANNOTATED FURTHER READING

Poulton, E.C. (1994). *Behavioural decision theory: A new approach.* Cambridge: Cambridge University Press.

An excellent introduction to the science of heuristics and the normative 'rules' that can be used to combat them … (or harness them where they are powerful). A little heavy for the non-psychologist but well worth the read.

Wulff, H.R. & Gotzsche, P.C. (2000). *Rational diagnosis and treatment: Evidence based clinical decision making (3rd edn).* London: Blackwell Science.

This introduces a number of key ideas that one should consider in diagnostic and treatment decisions (probably the fastest growing area of nurse decision making). The spectrum of disease, normative diagnostic process and Bayesian ideas applied to diagnosis are all covered.

Eddy, D.M. (1996). *Clinical decision making: From theory to practice.* Sudbury, MA: Jones and Bartlett.

A fantastic overview of the 'macro' problems associated with variable quality in professional decision making. Places many of the strategies discussed elsewhere in this book (such as guidelines) firmly in the context of the challenge to state provided health services which poor decisions represent.

REFERENCES

Arkes, H.R., Wortmann, R.L., Saville, P.D., & Harkness, A.R. (1966). Hindsight bias among physicians weighing the likelihood of diagnoses. *Journal of Applied Psychology, 3*, 252–254.

Benner, P. (1984). *From novice to expert: Excellence and power in clinical nursing practice.* Menlo Park, CA: Addison-Wesley.

Benner, P. & Tanner, C.A. (1987). Clinical judgement: How expert nurses use intuition. *American Journal of Nursing, 87*(1), 23–31.

Benner, P., Hooper-Kyriakidis, P., & Stannard, D. (1999). *Clinical wisdom and interventions in critical care: A thinking in action approach.* London: WB Saunders.

Christensen-Szalanski, B.J.B. (1981). Physicians' use of probabilistic information in a real clinical setting. *Journal of Experimental Psychology: Human Perception and Performance, 7*, 928–935.

Cioffi, J. (1997). Heuristics, servants to intuition, in clinical decision-making. *Journal of Advanced Nursing, 26*, 203–208.

Deutsch, T., Carson, E., & Ludwig, E. (1994). *Dealing with medical knowledge: Computers in clinical decision making.* New York: Plenum Press.

Dowie, J. & Elstein, A. (1988). *Professional judgement. A reader in clinical decision making.* Cambridge: Cambridge University Press.

Dreyfus, H.L. & Dreyfus, S.E. (1986). *Mind over machine: The power of human intuition and expertise in the era of the computer.* New York: Free Press.

Fischoff, B. (1975). Hindsight – foresight: the effect of outcome knowledge on judgement under uncertainty. *Journal of Experimental Psychology: Human Perception and Performance, 1*, 288–299.

Friedlander, M. & Stockman, S. (1983). Anchoring and publicity effects in clinical judgement. *Journal of Clinical Psychology, 39*, 637–643.

Gigerenzer, G. (1991). How to make cognitive illusions disappear: Beyond 'heuristics and biases'. *European Review of Social Psychology, 2*, 83–115.

Hammond, K.R. (1964). An approach to the study of clinical inference in nursing: Part II. *Nursing Research, 13*(4), 315–319.

Jones, P.R. (1995). Hindsight bias in reflective practice: An empirical investigation. *Journal of Advanced Nursing, 21*, 783–788.

Kahneman, D. & Tversky, A. (1973). On the psychology of prediction. *Psychological Review, 80*, 237–251.

Lichenstein, S. & Fischoff, B. (1977). Do those who know more also know more about how much they know? The calibration of probability judgements. *Organizational Behaviour and Human Performance, 20*, 159–183.

Poulton, E.C. (1994). *Behavioural decision theory: A new approach.* Cambridge: Cambridge University Press.

Reason, J. (1998). *Human error.* Cambridge: Cambridge University Press.

Royal College of Nursing (1998). *Clinical practice guidelines: the management of patients with venous leg ulcers.* London: Royal College of Nursing.

Simon, H.A. (1982). *Models of bounded rationality: Behavioural economics and business organisation.* Cambridge, MA: MIT Press.

Tversky, A. & Kahneman, P. (1973). Availability: A heuristic for judging frequency and probability. *Cognitive Psychology, 5*, 207–232.

3

What are clinical judgements?

Jane Cioffi

Observation tells us the fact, reflection the meaning of the fact.... The trained power of attending to one's own impressions made by one's own senses, so that these should tell the nurse how the patient is, is the sine qua non *of being a nurse.*
(Nightingale, 1907, pp. 254–255)

KEY ISSUES

◆ Clinical judgements feed clinical decisions and are just as prone to errors.

◆ Different judgement tasks merit different approaches to clinical judgement.

◆ Strategies to improving clinical judgements exist and can be applied by nurses in practice.

◆ Ways need to be explored to impart the judgement skills of the expert to (less experienced) novices in clinical practice.

Quality nursing care is dependent on good clinical decision making, which in turn is based on accurate judgements. According to Kritek (1985) and Jones (1988), the very least a patient should be able to expect, from a legal and ethical perspective, is an adequate description by nurses of the judgements that lead to decisions. As the above quote by Florence Nightingale highlights, one of the main foci of nursing judgement is the assessment of the patient. This focus on patient assessment and management of treatment is the crux of nursing judgement and has important implications for how decisions regarding treatment are made. This chapter examines the characteristics of judgement in nursing practice, including the strategies and thought processes used to make judgements and the role of experience in that process.

WHAT ARE CLINICAL JUDGEMENTS?

When discussing medical practice, it is fairly obvious that the main focus of practice is that of making a medical diagnosis (judgement) before deciding on appropriate treatment for the patient (decision). The main focus of practice in nursing is by its nature less obvious, and one of the central tasks for nurses and researchers alike to try and 'capture' the nature of judgement and decision making in nursing.

A number of studies have examined how nurses make judgements and decisions in practice. These studies suggest that the focus of nursing practice are issues such as identifying clinical deterioration, assessment of the patient's current and previous condition (Cioffi, 2000) and the prediction of future events (such as whether or not someone is likely to have a problem after theatre) (Cioffi, 1998). Therefore the core of nursing practice appears to be the management of patient problems and their treatment, not their diagnosis (Farrand et al., 1995; Holzemer, 1986).

A study carried out by Lamond et al. (1996) attempted to classify the types of judgements nurses made in acute medical and surgical ward environments. From interviews with 104 nurses they identified four different types of judgements that nurses made in practice (Box 3.1). Of these, descriptive and evaluative judgements were the most frequently used. The statements used to express these types of judgement included references to the severity of the patient's illness, the stability or instability of the patient's condition and the presence of pain. This is supported by another study by Lamond (2000), which found that descriptive and evaluative statements about patient care and condition were more likely to be communicated during the change of shift report. Another aspect of nursing judgement that is not highlighted in these research studies, but is evident in the *practice* of nursing, is that of prediction, which is often related to the 'risk' of something happening to a patient. This particular aspect of nursing judgement is covered in more detail in Chapter 5, so is not discussed further here.

In terms of how the typology of judgements compares to that of decision making in nursing, one of the most important aspects to be aware of is the nature of judgements: they are assessments of the patient state or condition (be it improved, the same or worse). Judgements can be used

---

Box 3.1 Types of judgements (from Lamond et al., 1996)

◆ Causal judgements (diagnosis)
   A statement expressing a state or condition based on the presence of attributes which are used to explain a problem.

◆ Descriptive judgements
   A statement expressing a state or condition based on the presence of attributes which had been observed directly or obtained from another source.

◆ Evaluative judgements
   A statement expressing a qualitative difference in a state or condition based on the presence of attributes which had been observed directly or obtained from another source.

◆ Inference judgements
   A statement expressing the presence of a state or condition which is not based on any information gathered from or about the patient.

> **Box 3.2** Examples of judgements leading to decisions (from Benner et al., 1996, pp. 126–127)
>
> *Around midnight he started getting a bit more pale [**judgement**]... and his lung sounds were okay [**judgement**]. ... by about 2 a.m. he was looking quite a bit worse and very wet [**judgement**]. ... So I got blood gas [**decision**] and the pH was 7.2. ... I finished giving the bicarb about a half hour previously and I looked at the baby and he looked much worse than he had before [**judgement**]. ... His mouth was just open slightly. He was gasping to try to breathe. He just looked awful, looked absolutely terrible [**judgement**]. ... So I gave the Lasix [**decision**], but at that point the baby was looking so bad [**judgement**] that I didn't even wait for the Lasix to take effect before I went ahead and did another blood gas [**decision**].*
>
> *Emphases added by author.*

as information to lead to another judgement or as an input into future decisions, as the example in Box 3.2 illustrates. Therefore issues such as how judgements are made, and their accuracy, are extremely important for practice. The rest of this chapter explores these issues in more detail.

THE CLINICAL JUDGEMENT PROCESS

Several different theoretical perspectives form the basis for investigating clinical judgement: information-processing theory, hermeneutics and decision analysis (or utility maximisation theory) (Fonteyn, 1995). Studies have conceptualised the clinical judgement process differently (e.g. hypothetico-deductive, concept attainment, pattern recognition and intuitive). The focus of these studies has been predominantly on patient assessment and the planning of care. Less attention has been given to the judgement process during the implementation of care and evaluations of the effectiveness of this care. In this section the results of these studies with regard to the types of strategies used by nurses and the accuracy of judgements are discussed.

Judgement tasks and strategies

Studies that have tried to describe the thought processes nurses use to make judgements have found that they often use a 'hypothetico-deductive' approach (see Ch. 1). Nurses use clinical information and knowledge to form single or multiple hypotheses that are predictive explanations of information. Studies show that in the generation of such hypotheses the strategies most frequently used are 'cue-based' (Tanner et al., 1987). The most commonly elicited cue is 'current state' (Corcoran-Perry & Graves, 1990; Gordon, 1980; Itano, 1989; Jacovone & Dostal, 1992). After hypotheses are generated they are tested through further inquiry, a process that Tanner et al. (1987) describe as 'iterative'. In tasks where information is potentially unlimited, multiple hypothesis testing decreases as progress is made towards attaining the state of the patient (Gordon, 1980).

Some reasoning strategies used in the judgement process have also been identified, namely, backward and forward reasoning (Cioffi, 1995). In forward reasoning an individual works forwards from the information given to find a problem solution. In backward reasoning an individual works backwards from a goal to evaluate different options or find a solution (Lamond et al., 1996). In conditions where the hypothetical (predicted) clinical state or plan of care fails to provide an explanation for new information, backward reasoning is used to search available data for support or substantiation of a clinical hunch. In conditions where new information is incorporated to further refine the view or plan held, a forward reasoning strategy is employed. Different reasoning strategies will be used in different situations.

Studies indicate that a wide range of strategies are used to make judgements and that these strategies are task-dependent (Benner, 1984; Benner & Tanner, 1987; Corcoran, 1986a, b; Gordon, 1980; Tanner et al., 1987). The judgement tasks of clinical practice, particularly in patient assessment situations, are often complex or uncertain (Kelly, 1964; Tanner, 1984; Tierney, 1987). When levels of uncertainty vary in assessment tasks, nurses rely on heuristic strategies or 'rules of thumb' such as the ones discussed in Chapter 2 (Cioffi, 1997, 1998). Reliance on such rules increases in frequency as the level of uncertainty heightens.

The heuristics used in task conditions of uncertainty involve assessments of probability (likelihood). Some evidence indicates that nurses use prior experiences in assessments of likelihood, for example, in clinical conditions with the potential to precipitate complications. This effect of causal significance is clearly seen in the overestimation of base rates by midwives for breech, threatened premature labour and antepartum haemorrhage (Cioffi, 1995). This is an example of the use of the representativeness heuristic, which requires previous experience with groups of similar cases. Another type of heuristic, 'availability', is found in the judgements of nurses and midwives in emergency and childbirth assessments (Cioffi, 1997, 1998). This heuristic is associated with recency of experience with a similar case and the salience or vividness of a particular clinical event in

> **Box 3.3** Use of propositional rules in reasoning
>
> The following example demonstrates the working form of a propositional rule:
>
> The categoric premise (e.g. child's temperature is 40°C) affirms the antecedent of the conditional premise (e.g. if child's temperature is 40°C) and the conclusion (e.g. then child may have convulsion) is a predictable outcome of the antecedent condition (Cioffi, 1998).
>
> *If* the child has a temperature of 40°C, *then* the child may have a convulsion.

memory and related to the presenting case. Clinical experience is associated with the development of heuristics, with more experienced nurses having larger repertoires of such heuristics (Cioffi, 1995).

Although heuristic strategies often result in reasonably valid judgements (optimal use) they can be associated with error or suboptimal use (Plous, 1993; Tversky & Kahneman, 1974), again as discussed in Chapter 2. Suboptimal use of the availability heuristic was found by Tanner (1977) in the judgement process of inexperienced nurses. Cioffi (1995) found optimal use of the representativeness, availability and anchoring and adjustment heuristics. Further investigation of the influence of heuristics on accuracy in judgements is required, because these findings are inconclusive.

Other studies have found nurses to use some propositional rules (If *X* is present then *Y* will occur) in their strategies to synthesise information (Cioffi, 1995; Gordon, 1980; Jacovone & Dostal, 1992; Marks et al., 1991). An example used by Gordon (1980) was '*If* it were the first or second day since surgery *then* suspect haemorrhagic shock or urinary retention'. These rules were used to combine cues, estimate likelihood and synthesise prior knowledge. Such rules can contain knowledge developed in clinical practice and are a valid form of argument that sets the stage for judgement. An example of this can be seen in Box 3.3. By applying rules stored in memory, knowledge is brought into the judgement process to make meaning of the presenting clinical situation.

Judgement accuracy

Factors found to contribute to inaccuracies in judgement all relate to how information is processed. Studies have shown that nurses can place too much reliance on a sign or a symptom that has little or no validity. Conversely, nurses can ignore cues of high validity (Kelly, 1964). Also, increasing amounts of information and involvement of information of low relevance result in error (Cianfrani, 1984; Hughes & Young, 1990). This issue is also discussed with regard to social judgement theory in Chapter 5.

Accuracy is also associated with experience, restricted amounts of data and (self-reported) high levels of confidence (Cioffi, 1995; Corcoran, 1986a; Gordon, 1980; Tanner, 1984, 1987). Individuals who have more experience are often more accurate, tasks with restricted amounts of data are linked to higher accuracy and higher levels of confidence are linked to greater accuracy. The early generation of a correct hypothetical judgement (Cianfrani, 1984; Gordon, 1989), and not testing multiple hypotheses involving contextual data (e.g. age, gender, surgery type) in the second half of the task, has also been found to contribute to accuracy (Gordon, 1980).

The use of models for shaping optimal judgements in the decision making process has been tried. To determine how models actually influence judgement performance, optimal judgements were developed and presented in a model of quantitative decision support for various postoperative situations requiring interventions (Hughes & Young, 1990). Nurses were found to agree with the predicted judgements of the model in conditions of lower uncertainty and to have diminished agreement in conditions of increased uncertainty. Models may be useful in clinical situations where certainty is high. However, they may be limited where conditions of uncertainty exist, for example, when patients have multiple pre-existing conditions and clinical problems.

The role of experience

Many studies have investigated the clinical judgement of nurses, with their subjective views providing valuable insight into the role experience plays in judgement (Agan, 1987; Benner, 1984; Benner & Tanner, 1987; Pyles & Stern, 1983; Schraeder & Fischer, 1987; Young, 1987). The common features that all these studies highlight is the importance of experience (with similar patients), 'knowing the patient' and judgement rules (similar to those discussed in the previous section). A common strand within these studies is the role that expertise plays in the judgement process.

Nurses seem to use past experiences when processing information about clinical situations. Their accounts of judging clinical deterioration to make decisions to call emergency support for patients reveal details of this process. Nurses talk of 'similar patients with a similar condition'. Some examples of this can be seen in Box 3.4. Another use of past experiences is built around causal significance associated with a patient condition/situation. In such situations, a nurse has had an experience where a particular outcome has occurred. The judgement is then based on the past experience of a probable outcome of the patient's presenting state (Baumann & Bourbonnais, 1982; Broderick & Ammentorp, 1979). Examples of this can also be found in Box 3.4. Here, the nurse is bringing the past experience to the current clinical situation to make meaning of the context and clinical information in order to form a judgement. This repeated exposure to similar events enable nurses to use the representativeness heuristic and memories of particular cases that are clinically vivid or recent – the availability heuristic.

Box 3.4 Examples of how past experience influences judgement

Similar patients with a similar condition

'You've looked after so many of them in a similar condition of CCF [congestive cardiac failure] that you know they are going to pulmonary oedema.' (Cioffi, 2000)

'… having worked with MIs [myocardial infarctions] and having observed what's their routine progression: how most of them recover. And seeing one that falls aside from that pattern, that's when I start getting worried … ' (Pyles & Stern, 1983)

Past experience of a probable outcome of the patient's presenting state

'What is happening now is a similar story to what happened to another particular patient. You think of the consequences of what happened to that previous patient and you think I need to keep a close eye on this for a while.' (Cioffi, 2000)

'This lady had just been seen by the medical officer and declared to be "fine" with orders to have her drain out and go home. When I went to take the drain out she was complaining of terrible pain, had quite bloodstained drainage and there was something not quite right. This lady went back to theatre. The other night a gentleman brought back memories of that incident as he also had bloodstained drainage.' (Cioffi, 2000)

Knowing the patient

'You can tell by looking at someone when you know them … you pick up on the little things. There are obvious signs that someone has deteriorated but a lot you pick up before they actually deteriorate.' (Cioffi, 2000)

(continued)

Box 3.4 *(continued)*

'Nothing was particularly wrong at the time but I just had a very bad feeling ... if you have been looking after them you can just tell.' *(Cioffi, 2000)*

'... some patients you have a sort of gut feeling ... their observations have not become compromised ... but you feel things are not quite right with them.' *(Cioffi, 2000)*

'The colour is not right ... a bit ... could be greyish not quite greyish as that is too far ... more sallow, pallid.' *(Cioffi, 2000)*

'Not feeling normal, no warmth, bit cool.' *(Cioffi, 2000)*

'The observations maybe a bit off though sometimes there is no change or only a marginal change present but there is something not right about them.' *(Cioffi, 2000)*

Rules

An emergency nurse triaging a male patient:

'If male with thin build then maybe a spontaneous pneumothorax.' *(Cioffi, 1998)*

A cardiovascular clinical nurse specialist:

'If systolic blood pressure 80 or below, the patient's blood is being directed to the vital organs and not the kidneys; therefore urine volume is decreased.' *(Cocoran-Perry & Graves, 1992)*

Midwives:

'If baby presenting in posterior position then labour will be longer.' *(Cioffi, 1995)*

'If presenting part is soft and irregular maybe a breech.' *(Cioffi, 1995)*

In judging clinical deterioration nurses may also refer to 'knowing the patient'. Examples of this type of use of experience can also be found in Box 3.4. The relevance of this characteristic for making judgements has been supported by other studies (Jenny & Logan, 1992; Radwin, 1996; Tanner et al., 1993). Nurses have described sensing or feeling that something is wrong, sometimes referring to this as a hunch, sixth sense or gut feeling. The cues described in these accounts of the judgement process are being perceptually measured. Judgements such as 'something going on' and 'not quite right' lead to decisions to call the medical emergency team (Cioffi, 2000). Nurses in such situations are aware of personal feelings, like a 'personal barometer' picking up subjective aspects of situations.

Nurses also talk of patients recognising differences in themselves and then conveying them to nurses (Benner, 1984; Benner & Tanner, 1987;

Orme & Maggs, 1993; Pyles & Stern, 1983; Young, 1987). Similarly, nurses describe differences they observe and judge in patients. For example, skin colour, temperature and observations when picking up clinical deterioration. Such descriptions show judgements of qualitative distinctions that in some cases are ratings of the degree to which something is present or not present in the patient. This enables partially useful information to be used rather than discarded. In the examples in Box 3.4, one of the nurses demonstrates the process of using an initial value (e.g. 'normal observations') and then adjusting it to form a judgement (e.g. 'maybe a bit off'). This is a verbal estimate of probability and an example of the use of the 'anchoring and adjustment' heuristic.

Sometimes the knowledge used in making judgements comes from rules similar to the propositional rules described earlier (Box 3.4). These rules are domain specific and it is expected that nurses hold sets of such procedural rules, which they access from memory to make meaning of clinical situations.

All of the studies examined highlight that making judgements is a continuous, rather than discrete, event. The process includes: using rules and prior experiences as support and as rationales, knowing the patient, gut feelings or an equivalent non-specific feeling that something is 'different' or 'not right'. Judgement involves the perception of qualitative distinctions in the patient and picking up differences that are reported by patients themselves.

Expertise in judgement

According to Pyles and Stern (1983), previous clinical experience is important in developing judgement skills. Experienced and inexperienced nurses have been found to have significantly different judgement process rating scores. This gap supports the idea of broad novice–expert differences in the judgement process (Itano, 1989). Other studies have identified the specific nature of these differences.

One of the main differences between expert and novice practitioners lies in their use of information when making judgements. Experience appears to influence nurse's information collection strategies and how they focus and adapt the search to the task conditions. Experts seem to be able to identify how relevant the information is, using forward reasoning and referring to past experience when making judgements. This is reflected in the number of cues experienced nurses collect, although the types of cues that they use compared to novices are essentially in the same proportion. Previous experiences with similar conditions are used to direct their information search and focus on relevant symptoms (Jacovone & Dostal, 1992). Experienced nurses view clinical elements separately (Jacovone & Dostal, 1992) and regard only parts of the clinical information as relevant. They also spread their search very quickly over a wide range of possibilities, thereby activating, accepting or rejecting a complex series of related categories. This is highlighted by the generation of more cognitively complex hypotheses than those generated by inexperienced nurses (Westfall et al., 1986), and the predominant use of forward reasoning (Cioffi, 1995). Overall, experienced nurses make judgements faster and more accurately than inexperienced nurses (Cioffi, 1995; Corcoran, 1986a; Tanner, 1984), a feature thought to be related to the highly structured knowledge base in an experienced nurse's long term memory.

Inexperienced nurses are less able to consider a wide range of factors in their search strategies (Broderick & Ammentorp, 1979; Corcoran, 1986a). They use whatever information is opportune in all cases, regardless of complexity (Corcoran, 1986a), and consider all parts of the clinical picture to be equally relevant. Within their reasoning process they do not reflect on past experiences, use mainly propositional knowledge learned in context-free situations (Benner, 1984) and often rely on backward reasoning (Cioffi, 1995). They bias their judgements by underestimating the value of disconfirming information and overestimating the value of confirmatory information, especially when only one active hypothesis is being tested (Matthews & Gaul, 1981; Tanner, 1977). These characteristics restrict the ability of less experienced nurses in their judgement processes, and are thought to be due to having less well organised ways of structuring knowledge in their long term memory.

LIMITATIONS IN JUDGEMENT RESEARCH

The fragmented nature of studies addressing aspects of the clinical judgement process has not yet resulted in a comprehensive understanding of the phenomenon. Consequently its effect on guiding nurses to achieve more accurate judgements has been minimal. What is known reflects the descriptive approaches taken by studies. The complexity in clinical situations, for example, patients with multiple coexisting conditions, most often make the study of the judgement process difficult and the identification of strategies to support more effective judgement a challenge.

Studies using a descriptive approach frequently use information processing theory to explore the ways in which nurses actually make judgements. This approach has contributed more to understanding the cognitive process involved, particularly in assessment and, to a lesser degree, planning. The ecological validity of such studies has been questioned (Gordon, 1972; Greenwood & King, 1995; Tanner et al., 1987). Criticism has focused predominantly on the representativeness of the judgement tasks used. In particular, there is the possibility that responses elicited are not like those that occur in actual practice (Tanner et al., 1987), and that making judgements away from the clinical setting may not induce the same cognitive strain and commensurate effect on accuracy (Gordon, 1972).

Accuracy is critical to good clinical judgement and it is essential that studies focus on this aspect in the future. To date, only a small number of factors have been associated with judgement error and sources of systematic error in the judgement process need to be explored. Studies in other disciplines have identified these sources of systematic error and the limits they place on judgements (Dawson & Arkes, 1987). Examples of such influences are seeking out only confirmatory information, ignoring negative evidence and the effects of framing.

Studies reviewed have methodological limitations, such as their poor ecological validity and potential for generalisation. Some of the findings, however, have been confirmed by other studies, which suggests they can provide some insight and understanding of the judgement process. It is time to find ways to make contributions of lasting value to the examination of judgement in nursing and midwifery practice. This could include considering new approaches, such as the theory of information integration (Anderson, 1991), or exploring differences in knowledge structures of experienced and less experienced nurses. By identifying experienced skilled nurses and examining their judgement in specific practice areas it may be possible to explore search strategies that identify critical data for making particular judgements, identify relationships between task characteristics and types of strategies, and determine strategies that are accurate and time efficient.

SOME TIPS FOR IMPROVING JUDGEMENT IN PRACTICE

In clinical judgement situations, nurses are most likely to apply strategies that are appropriate to the degree of certainty of information available. In actual clinical practice, elements of the clinical information available are quite certain (e.g. temperature) and others less certain (e.g. general malaise). Some judgements are based on certainty and others on uncertainty. More certainty enables more 'rational' judgements to be formed due to the reduced number of alternatives from which to select. Less certainty requires nurses to use a more probabilistic approach to their judgements. In these estimations of probability or likelihood, with their incomplete and low levels of relevant data derived from prior experiences, there is potential for error. Nurses can therefore actively strengthen their judgement processes by applying some simple checks. Checking your own judgement process can make you more aware of how you form judgements. This section discusses aspects of the judgement process you might like to reflect on and offers some suggestions for you to try.

Reliance on memory

As your mind is unable to keep track of all the data you collect, you take short cuts to arrive at judgements. From the knowledge stored in your memory you access similar situations, cases and events, or a particular example you have experienced, and use them to make sense of the presenting clinical situation. Inherent in working in this way are personal biases. These biases – systematic tendencies – are born of experience and represent your preferences for given conclusions or inferences over other possible alternatives.

Nurses have their own personal set of clinical experiences to draw on. They need to be cognisant of these when examining influences on the judgements they are forming. Recollections of memories used in this way are based, for example, on the vividness, salience or recency of a particular case or a group of similar patients. Box 3.5 summarises the common strategies we use to limit our need for processing, and some strategies you could try to combat them.

Estimating probabilities

Nurses use words that are qualitatively distinct to communicate patient information. Words such as 'likely', 'maybe', 'probably', 'could be', are used when communicating judgements about patients that can lead to decisions. These words are verbal estimates of probability or likelihood and can create serious misunderstanding and error. Different interpretations of these words can result in wide variations in what is understood. To check the degree of consistency that is held for these estimations among other nurses with whom you work, you might like to consider translating them into numerical probabilities (e.g. 0.8 or 80%) and comparing assigned values.

Box 3.5 Influences of memory and strategies

Memory effects on judgement

◆ Recalling a particular case based on the ease with which it comes to mind.

◆ Seeing a goodness of fit between the presenting, and previously experienced, cases based on piece after piece of information being consistent with what you are considering.

◆ Adjusting values from an initial point too much or not enough.

◆ Seeing more potency in causal information than in non-causal information.

Strategies to try

◆ Looking for what does not fit rather than what fits.

◆ Reframing by shifting perspective; for example, 'how inactive is the patient?' can be shifted to 'how active is the patient?'.

◆ Reviewing causal attribution.

◆ Respecting ambiguity in the data by continuing to remain open rather than closing off too quickly.

◆ Considering reasons why you may be incorrect.

Often, statements such as 'quite restless' or 'some anxiety' are used at shift handover or in written reports. These judgements are estimations that are based on a nurse's own personal rating scale for estimating the degree of presence of these clinical entities in patients. They also are open to interpretation and, without observing the described difference, difficult to understand. Ideally, additional description to indicate what has led to this estimation should be documented or explained. To provide a clearer appreciation of the patient's status it may be useful to actually go to the bedside of the patient and assess the patient together.

In some instances it is possible to use available information presented in texts, journals and national or local databases, rather than personal experience when estimating probability or risk. Compiling databases for adverse occurrences in your clinical populations from case records can be useful for building better evidence on which to base judgements. For example, what is the risk of a patient who has had a particular procedure for a particular adverse occurrence (e.g. decubitus ulcer) based on its occurrence in your ward? This can have implications for making decisions about the nursing care this type of patient may require, reducing the risk of an adverse occurrence. Benchmarking your local outcomes by comparing rates for adverse occurrences with national statistics can identify marked differences and can help identify local contributory factors to the differences observed.

Peer evaluation of adverse occurrences

By using peer review of cases with adverse patient occurrences attributable to nursing practice, the judgement process can be reviewed and areas that are open to improvement discussed. To improve the judgement process this form of quality monitoring needs to be non-punitive. It needs to be focused on practice that nurses are legally responsible for, to have clearly outlined procedural guidelines for each review and be outcome oriented.

Development of judgement skills

Judgements made in clinical practice are not overt aspects of practice – strategies can be incorporated into practice to make them more explicit. Judgements are context specific and nurses with more experience in particular practice domains could consider ways to support the development of judgement skills in less experienced nurses. When opportunities occur in daily practice and where judgement is an issue, nurses can discuss (in an open and constructive manner) how they form their judgements in order to enhance already existing skills. The discussion of rules used by experienced nurses to arrive at their judgements may also be of value.

Another useful strategy for gaining additional skills for a specific clinical role, such as triaging patients in emergency departments, is the use of simulations and 'thinking aloud' (Cioffi, 1999). Simulations based on cases from practice can be developed to provide clinical situations in which the judgement process can be coached. In such simulations nurses can 'talk aloud' the thought processes they are using to collect and synthesise the information.

CONCLUSION

The purpose of this chapter was to provide you with an overview of the main issues of concern when considering clinical judgement in nursing. As has been discussed, there is a need for more research into the accuracy of judgements and how to improve judgement in nursing. An understanding of how important clinical judgements are in nursing and midwifery practice, in terms of how they feed the decisions we make about patient care, is important if we are to provide patients with good quality health care.

QUESTIONS FOR DISCUSSION

◆ What are the common judgements you make in practice?

◆ How might these be improved?

◆ Think of someone you consider to be a clinical 'expert'. Does he or she make good clinical judgements? Why? How can this person's skills be disseminated throughout the entire team?

ANNOTATED FURTHER READING

Benner, P., Hooper-Kyriakidis, P., & Stannard, D. (1999). *Clinical wisdom and interventions in critical care. A thinking-in-action approach.* Philadelphia: WB Saunders.

The concepts laid out in this book will resonate with all who face clinical thinking in dynamic patient care situations. The authors illustrate 'thinking-in-action' and 'reasoning-in-transition' in real practice situations. Six aspects of clinical judgement and skillful comportment are highlighted in each domain to guide active reflection on practice as a means to capture the nature of expert clinical judgement and comportment.

Fonteyn, M.E. (1998). *Thinking strategies for nursing practice.* Philadelphia: Lippincott.

This book is based on a descriptive study of nurses' thinking in practice. Twelve predominant thinking strategies found to be consistently used by nurse participants are described and accompanied by numerous clinical examples. The final section of the book focuses on how nurses think when resolving clinical dilemmas. A variety of thinking activities are included to assist the reader to develop effective thinking strategies.

Goldstein, W.M. & Hogarth, R.M. (eds) (1997). *Research on judgement and decision making. Currents, connections and controversies.* Cambridge: Cambridge University Press.

This book presents an overview of recent research on the psychology of judgement and decision making. The three sections – currents, connections and controversies – contain significant recent papers. In the 'currents' section, topics such as acquisition and use of knowledge and causal judgement are addressed and in 'connections', memory and explanation and judgement. Finally, in 'controversies', domain knowledge, content specificity, rule-governed versus rule-described behaviour are among the topics discussed.

Higgs, J. & Jones, M. (eds) (1995). *Clinical reasoning in health professions.* Oxford: Butterworth-Heinemann.

This book presents clinical reasoning as thinking and decision making processes which are integral to clinical practice. The nature of clinical reasoning and the development of clinical reasoning expertise are discussed, followed by an examination of clinical reasoning in the practice of medicine, nursing, physiotherapy and occupational therapy. The remaining part of the book focuses on the teaching of clinical reasoning with emphasis on an adult learning approach.

Manktelow, K. (1999). *Reasoning and thinking.* East Sussex: Psychology Press.

This book reviews psychological research in the areas of reasoning and thinking – deduction, induction, hypothesis testing, probability judgement and decision making – and covers the major theoretical debates in the area.

REFERENCES

Agan, R.D. (1987). Intuitive knowing as a dimension of nursing. *Advances in Nursing Science, 10*(1), 63–70.

Anderson, N.H. (1991). A cognitive theory of judgement and decision. In: Anderson, N.H. (ed.), *Contributions to information integration theory. Volume 1. Cognition* (pp. 105–142). New Jersey: Lawrence Erlbaum.

Baumann, A. & Bourbonnais, F. (1982). Nursing decision making in critical care. *Journal of Advanced Nursing, 7*, 435–446.

Benner, P. (1984). *From novice to expert: Excellence and power in clinical nursing practice.* Menlo Park, CA: Addison-Wesley.

Benner, P. & Tanner, C.A. (1987). Clinical judgment: How expert nurses use intuition. *American Journal of Nursing, 87*(1), 23–31.

Benner, P., Tanner, C.A., & Chelsa, C.A. (1996). *Expertise in nursing practice: caring, clinical judgment, and ethics.* New York: Springer.

Broderick, M.E. & Ammentorp, W. (1979). Information structures: An analysis of nursing performance. *Nursing Research, 28*(2), 106–110.

Cianfrani, K.L. (1984). The influence of amounts and relevance of data on identifying health problems. In: Kim, M.J., McFarlane, G.K., & McLane, A.M. (eds), *Classification of nursing diagnoses: Proceedings of the fifth national conference* (pp. 150–161). St Louis: Mosby.

Cioffi, J. (1995). *The effect of uncertainty on heuristic use by nurses in patient assessment situations.* Doctoral dissertation, University of Sydney.

Cioffi, J. (1997). Heuristics, servants to intuition, in clinical decision-making. *Journal of Advanced Nursing, 26,* 203–208.

Cioffi, J. (1998). Decision making by emergency nurses. *Accident and Emergency Nursing, 6,* 184–191.

Cioffi, J. (1999). Triage decision making: Educational strategies. *Accident and Emergency Nursing, 7*(2), 106–111.

Cioffi, J. (2000). Nurses' experiences of making decisions to call emergency assistance to their patients. *Journal of Advanced Nursing, 32*(1), 108–114.

Corcoran, S.A. (1986a). Planning by expert and novice nurses in cases of varying complexity. *Research in Nursing and Health, 9,* 155–162.

Corcoran, S.A. (1986b). Task complexity and nursing expertise as factors in decision making. *Nursing Research, 35*(2), 107–112.

Corcoran-Perry, S. & Graves, J. (1990). Supplemental-information-seeking behavior of cardiovascular nurses. *Research in Nursing and Health, 13,* 119–127.

Dawson, N.V. & Arkes, H.R. (1987). Systematic errors in medical decision making: Judgement limitations. *Journal of General Internal Medicine, 2,* 183–187.

Farrand, L., Leprohon, J., Kalina, M., Champagne, F., Contandriopoulos, A.P., & Preker, A. (1995). The role of protocols and professional judgement in emergency medical dispatching. *European Journal of Emergency Medicine, 2*(3), 136–148.

Fonteyn, M. (1995). Clinical reasoning in nursing. In: Higgs, J. & Jones, M. (eds), *Clinical reasoning in the health professions.* Oxford: Butterworth-Heinemann.

Gordon, M. (1972). *Strategies in probabilistic concept attainment. A study of nursing diagnosis.* Doctoral dissertation, Boston College, Massachusetts.

Gordon, M. (1980). Predictive strategies in diagnostic tasks. *Nursing Research, 29,* 39–45.

Gordon, M. (1989). Strategies for teaching diagnostic reasoning. In: Carroll-Johnson, R. (ed.), *Classification of nursing diagnosis: Proceedings of the eighth national conference* (pp. 43–49). Philadelphia: Lippincott.

Greenwood, J. & King, M. (1995). Some surprising similarities in the clinical reasoning of 'expert' and 'novice' orthopaedic nurses: Report of a study using verbal protocols and protocol analyses. *Journal of Advanced Nursing, 22,* 907–913.

Holzemer, W.L. (1986). The structure of problem solving in simulations. *Nursing Research, 35,* 231–236.

Hughes, K. & Young, W. (1990). The relationship between task complexity and decision making consistency. *Research in Nursing and Health, 13,* 189–197.

Itano, J.K. (1989). A comparison of the clinical judgment process in experienced registered nurses and student nurses. *Journal of Nursing Education, 28*(3), 120–126.

Jacovone, J. & Dostal, M. (1992). A descriptive study of nursing judgement in the assessment and management of cardiac pain. *Advances in Nursing Science, 15*(1), 54–63.

Jenny, J. & Logan, J. (1992). Knowing the patient: One aspect of clinical knowledge. *IMAGE: Journal of Nursing Scholarship, 24*(4), 254–258.

Jones, J.A. (1988). Clinical reasoning in nursing. *Journal of Advanced Nursing, 13*(2), 185–192.

Kelly, K.J. (1964). An approach to the study of clinical inference in nursing. Part 1. Introduction to the study of clinical inference in nursing. *Nursing Research, 23,* 314–315.

Kritek, P.B. (1985). Nursing diagnosis in perspective: Response to a critique. *IMAGE: Journal of Nursing Scholarship, 18*(1), 3–8.

Lamond, D. (2000). The information content of the nurse change of shift report: A comparative study. *Journal of Advanced Nursing, 31*(4), 794–804.

Lamond, D., Crow, R., & Chase, J. (1996). Judgements and processes in care decisions in acute medical and surgical wards. *Journal of Evaluation in Clinical Practice, 2*(3), 211–216.

Marks, R.J., Simons, R.S., Blizzard, R.A., & Browne, D.R.G. (1991). Predicting outcome in intensive therapy units – a comparison of APACHE II with subjective assessments. *Intensive Care Medicine, 17,* 159–163.

Matthews, C.A. & Gaul, A.L. (1981). Nursing diagnosis from the perspective of concept attainment. *Advances in Nursing Science, 1,* 17–26.

Nightingale, F. (1907). Training of nurses. In: Nutting, M.A. & Dock, A. (eds), *History of nursing, Volume 2*. New York: Putman & Sons.

Orme, L. & Maggs, C. (1993). Decision making in clinical practice: How do expert nurses, midwives and health visitors make decisions? *Nurse Education Today, 13*, 270–276.

Plous, S. (1993). *The psychology of judgement and decision making*. Philadelphia: Temple University Press.

Pyles, S.H. & Stern, P.N. (1983). Discovery of nursing gestalt in critical care nursing: The importance of the gray gorilla syndrome. *Image: The Journal of Nursing Scholarship, 15*(2), 51–57.

Radwin, L.E. (1996). 'Knowing the patient': A review of research on an emerging concept. *Journal of Advanced Nursing, 23*, 1142–1146.

Schraeder, B.D. & Fischer, D.K. (1987). Using intuitive knowledge in the neonatal intensive care nursery. *Holistic Nursing Practice, 1*(3), 45–51.

Tanner, C.A. (1977). *The effect of hypothesis generation as an instructional method on the diagnostic processes of senior baccalaureate nursing students*. Doctoral dissertation, University of Colorado, Boulder.

Tanner, C.A. (1984). Factors influencing the diagnostic process. In: Carnevali, D.L., Mitchell, P.H., Woods, N.F., & Tanner, C.A. (eds), *Diagnostic reasoning in nursing* (pp. 61–82). Philadelphia: Lippincott.

Tanner, C.A. (1987). Teaching clinical judgement. In: Fitzpatrick, J.J. & Taunton, R.L. (eds), *Annual review of nursing research, vol. 5* (pp. 153–173). New York: Springer.

Tanner, C.A., Padrick, K.P., Westfall, U.E., & Putzer, D.J. (1987). Diagnostic reasoning strategies of nurses and nursing students. *Nursing Research, 36*(6), 358–363.

Tanner, C.A., Benner, P., Chelsa, C., & Gordon, D.R. (1993). The phenomenology of knowing the patient. *IMAGE: Journal of Nursing Scholarship, 25*(4), 273–280.

Tierney, A.J. (1987). A view on clinical judgement and decision making from the perspective of the nursing process. *Clinical judgement and decision making: The future with nursing diagnosis. Proceedings of the international nursing conference* (pp. 260–267). New York: John Wiley & Sons.

Tversky, A. & Kahneman, D. (1974). Judgement under uncertainty: Heuristics and biases. *Science, 185*, 1124–1131.

Westfall, U.E., Tanner, C.A., Putzier, D., & Padrick, K.P. (1986). Activating clinical inferences. A component of diagnostic reasoning in nursing. *Research in Nursing and Health, 9*, 269–277.

Young, C. (1987). Intuition and the nursing process. *Holistic Nursing Practice, 1*(3), 52–56.

4

How nurses use clinical information in practice

Maxine Offredy

KEY ISSUES

- Clinical information used in decision making and judgement varies according to the situation faced.
- Using clinical information in decision making demands strategies which suit the varied nature of information types.
- Using clinical cues and other forms of information can be improved.

Expanding healthcare knowledge, new health technologies and new interventions all mean that modern nursing practice is becoming increasingly complex. These challenges raise issues regarding the clinical information nurses use to inform their practice. This chapter explores some of these issues and suggests ways to improve the use of information provided in practice. The chapter begins by exploring clinical information, what it is and what information nurses use in practice. Tips for how you can use information more effectively in your practice are also incorporated.

WHAT IS CLINICAL INFORMATION?

Often called clinical cues, forceful features or clinical data, clinical information refers to the data used by healthcare professionals and patients to make judgements and decisions about health care. For the purposes of this chapter, clinical information is defined as that quantitative (statistical, objective) and/or qualitative (intuitive, objective, subjective) data used by nurses to make diagnostic, therapeutic or management decisions. Clinical information can come from a number of sources. Table 4.1 provides some examples of different types of clinical information.

Nurses use a variety of different types of clinical information when making judgements and decisions in practice. For example, Lamond et al. (1996) investigated the sources of information registered nurses in acute medical and surgical wards use when making assessment judgements. They identified four main sources of information used by nurses: verbal communication, observation, prior knowledge and written material. These four areas were further subdivided into specific sources of information. The study found that the frequency with which verbal data was mentioned as a source of information was more than double that of observation, prior knowledge and written information (they were used 41, 21, 20 and 17% respectively). Further analysis of the data showed both medical and surgical nurses appearing to use verbal and written information to similar degrees. Surgical nurses used observation (visual cues) and prior knowledge (which could be both research and opinion based) slightly more than medical nurses.

In another study, Luker and Kenrick (1992) explored the factors influencing community nurses' decision making identifying 35 sources of influence. These were practice based knowledge ($n = 20$), common sense knowledge ($n = 3$), mixed research based/practice based knowledge ($n = 6$), research based ($n = 3$), with three unable to be classified. The nurses reported that practice based knowledge, the situational context

Table 4.1 Types and sources of clinical information

Type of clinical information	Source of clinical information
Qualitative: patients' perspectives of their condition	This refers to history taking of the patient's condition and involves a patient focused element where the nurse enters the patient's world to see the illness from the latter's perspective. By actively listening to what the patient has to say, cues are followed up by the nurse when the patient has the history giving explanation. Cues are salient pieces of information that help to provide an overall picture of the presenting problem. The central issue of patient focused history taking is to allow as much information as possible to flow from the patient
Qualitative: nurses' perspectives of a patient's condition	Nurses' perspectives of a patient's condition have been highlighted in a number of studies (Luker & Kenrick, 1992, Hallett et al., 2000, Lamond, 2000). These studies utilised nurses' experiences and knowledge to show how a decision was formulated about a patient's condition
Qualitative and quantitative: patient examination	Data gathered from patient examination may be subject to error, for example, the patient might state a symptom but the nurse could hear something else
Quantitative: laboratory results	White et al. (1992) studied 27 nurse practitioners in two different settings. They found that the nurses ordered the correct laboratory test necessary for a correct diagnosis but that they did not understand what the results indicated. This implied that choosing what information to obtain and then deciding on the intervention involved two different bodies of knowledge
Quantitative and qualitative: ambiguity of clinical information	Weinstein et al. (1980, p. 2) suggested that 'Information obtained by physical examination or a diagnostic procedure may be intrinsically ambiguous and may thus be interpreted differently by different observers'. This means that, when faced with the same information, variation can occur between patients and nurses can differ in their ability to detect the variations. The propensity to record exactly what has been observed or found varies between nurses. Further, nurses might apply different perceptual thresholds in deciding whether or not a clinical sign (a cue) is present or absent
Qualitative and quantitative: relationship between clinical information and the presence of disease	Patients differ in the degree of clinical signs and symptoms they manifest, even for the same common illnesses. A degree of uncertainty remains about the presence or absence of a clinical sign for even the most unambiguous of cases

and discussions with colleagues played a large part in their decision making process. Scientific knowledge was reported as being associated with the results of published research in nursing and medical journals and information from drug representatives. Only two participants were able to articulate reasons for their decisions. The evidence from the study suggests that nurses gave visual and subjective cues greater weight in their decision making processes than textual and objective data (the 'evidence'). The latter were less likely to find accommodation within the nurses' practice (they reported that only three out of the 35 influences on the decision making process were research based). However, the study made the point that scientific knowledge might have been incorporated in nursing knowledge and further reference to the primary source is not acknowledged. Thus the 20 sources of influence referred to as practice based knowledge may include reclassified scientific knowledge.

What these studies highlight is the variety of different sources of information that nurses use to inform their judgement and decision making in practice. This information is a mixture of previous knowledge (an issue also raised in Ch. 3) and more subjective and objective clinical signs.

IDENTIFYING INFORMATION

As well as considering the information nurses use when making judgements and decisions, you also need to consider how that information is identified. Hammond et al. (1966) examined the type of information seeking strategies nurses use when given a decision task. They examined the order in which information was selected by ten nurses, together with the value of the information to the nurse. They found that nurses used a variety of different types of strategy to search for relevant clinical information, which can be found in Box 4.1.

When confronted with a patient problem or condition, nurses attend selectively to information with a view to forming hypotheses for testing (see Ch. 1 for a description of this hypothetico-deductive approach to reasoning). Decisions are made about what information to collect, in what order and how the information will be used. Several studies (Bryans & McIntosh, 1996; Hallett, et al., 2000; Lamond, 2000; Lamond, et al., 1996; Marsden, 1999) explore the ways nurses make decisions and the data they elicit when making their judgements.

Marsden's (1999) investigation into telephone triage was undertaken in an ophthalmic accident and emergency department. The study sought

Box 4.1 Information seeking strategies

◆ *Simultaneous scanning strategy* – assessing information simultaneously to test multiple hypotheses based upon what has been chosen.

◆ *Successive scanning* – searching systematically for one piece of information at a time.

◆ *Ordering* – the order in which cues were selected. Four sets of ordering assumptions can be made:

  − selection

  − probability

  − successive scanning

  − simultaneous scanning orderings.

to explore whether knowledge of the decision making processes of nurse practitioners (NP) would assist in informing the practice and training of future nurses wishing to undertake the triaging role. Telephone triage decisions are slightly different from other forms of nurse decision making as decisions are made on the basis of the information elicited without seeing the patient (or the person making the telephone call). This means that the clinical information available to the nurse in telephone triage is more restricted (as visual information is not available). Using semi-structured interviews, the research elicited a range of signs and symptoms on which nurses' decisions were based. These provided both a mental picture of the patient and a provisional diagnosis of what might be wrong. Further clinical information was obtained confirming or refuting the early diagnosis. Nurses reported making provisional diagnoses at varying stages of the telephone conversation. Some participants identified significant pieces of clinical information in the telephone conversation, which led to the nurse giving the patient access to the service. These cues included excessive pain and recent loss of vision.

Hallett et al. (2000) looked at wound care decision making by community nurses. Semi-structured interviews were carried out with 62 nurses, focusing on successful encounters with patients and situations where difficulties had been experienced. This study found that thorough assessment was central to the nurses' encounter with patients. Factors that affected the nurses' judgement included: patient nutritional status, degree of mobility, weight, general wellbeing, attitude of the patient and the likelihood of treatment concordance.

What these studies highlight is the importance of knowledge, experience, questioning skills and knowing what information to ask the patient when making decisions. It is clear from these two studies that nurses seek, and use, a variety of cues in their decision making processes. These included the recognition of signs and symptoms en route to the construction of a mental picture of the condition, alongside further information from the patient to assist or reject provisional hypotheses. Moreover, whilst both subjective and objective data were used to reach decisions, it is clear that intuition is a key part of the nurses' decision making armoury. Russo and Schoemaker (1991) warn that the negative implications of using intuitive decision making are more profound than most people realise: intuition based decisions are far less reliable than they suspect (see Ch. 2). So, having established what cues nurses seek and use, the question now becomes, 'How do they use them?'

HOW DO NURSES USE CLINICAL INFORMATION?

This section focuses on the use of clinical information and the weighting, or importance, given to each piece of information in the process of forming a decision. The relative importance of the information selected probably differs in different circumstances and may be largely unknown to the decision maker. Knowledge of weightings, however, is accumulated incrementally. Namely, as patients seen in the past and recalled from memory become sufficiently numerous and accessible, a more reliable form of database is formed.

Decision tasks have been classified according to whether or not they are structured and their degree of complexity (Hammond, 1978). The more complex the problem, the more pieces of information will be elicited from the patient. Patients often present with a vague problem and the nurse needs to collect a number of cues in order to structure and order the decision problem. Furthermore, cues have a multiplicity of values and different levels of significance according to whether or not they are presented alone or combined with other cues. For example, consider Scenarios 4.1 and 4.2:

Scenario 4.1

Blood pressure reading of 150/85 mmHg in a 30-year-old Afro-Caribbean male on first visiting his GP practice.

Scenario 4.2

Blood pressure reading of 150/85 mmHg in a 30-year-old Afro-Caribbean male on first visiting his GP practice, rising to 160/85 after 10 minutes and producing the same reading after rechecking for a third time 30 minutes after his arrival.

In both scenarios the initial blood pressure reading may give cause for concern. In Scenario 4.1 the relatively high blood pressure reading in a young, healthy Afro-Caribbean male may mean that he is feeling anxious on first attending the surgery. In Scenario 4.2 the different blood pressure readings could be due to a number of causes, one of which could be family history; both, however, are just probable causes. Probability is measured on a scale from 0 to 1, where a certain cause or event is assigned a probability of 1 and an impossible cause or event is given a probability of 0. As has already been discussed in Chapter 2, in health care practice you can never be 100% sure of the outcome so the probability will never be 1. Phrases such as, 'usually ...', 'eight out of ten cases show that ...', 'nearly all participants had a reaction to ...' are all common expressions of this uncertainty.

The role uncertainty plays in information use in nursing practice is highlighted in a study by Cioffi (2000) investigating registered nurses' experiences of calling the medical emergency team (MET). Examples of uncertainty when calling included whether or not the nurses were doing the right thing and seeking the confirmatory opinions of their peers when uncertainty arose about the patient's 'fit' with the criteria for calling the MET. The study showed that the MET criteria outlined clinically objective stages of deterioration, but the nurses gave great weight to subjective data and pattern matching when recognising patients in the early stages of deterioration. Having previous knowledge of the patient was also a critical factor in making decisions about those at risk. Experience and complex clinical judgements appear inexorably linked in this study. Despite the importance of intuitive judgements, the nurses justified their call with objective data, even if this meant delaying the call until the patient met the criteria for calling the MET. Thus more emphasis or weight was placed on objective than subjective data when calling for medical assistance.

The above study shows that it is not easy to isolate the weighting placed on different cues by nurses. In addition, not all cues were articulated, leading to difficulties when attempting to explain how cues are used in decision making. In all cases, experience was an influential component in the nurses' decision making processes. Relying solely on experience can lead to nurses falling prey to 'decision traps' in their cognition (Russo & Schoemaker, 1991). There are two decision traps in this case:

◆ Over confidence in one's judgement – whereby insufficient key factual information has been collected because the decision maker is too confident in their own assumptions and opinions.
◆ 'Shooting from the hip' – believing that all the information pertaining to a particular case can be kept in one's head, is representative and that the 'rule of thumb' principle (see Ch. 2) should be followed instead of a systematic procedure.

AN EXAMPLE: DECISION MAKING IN ACTION

This example is taken from a much larger study addressing diagnostic and therapeutic decision making by nurse practitioners in primary care. The study involved 11 general practitioner (GP) and 11 nurse practitioner (NP) dyads (linked pairs). Six patient scenarios – text and photographic – were used. Reference models were devised for each scenario, allowing comparison of the practitioner responses. The scenarios were conditions or problems deemed suitable for consultation by either practitioner. Each practitioner was reminded of the aims of the study and of the 'think aloud' (Ericsson & Simon, 1993) procedure. Briefly, this procedure requires participants to verbalise their thoughts, i.e. to 'think aloud', regarding their plans for the patient.

The study was designed to examine both the judgement (making a diagnosis) and decision (deciding on a treatment intervention) processes in nurse practitioners and doctors and comparing their performance. Analysis of the thought processes of the participants was based around the four major stages of clinical reasoning identified by Elstein et al. (1978) and already discussed in Chapter 1.

A brief description of the scenario appears in Scenario 4.3, and an overview of the judgement and decision processes of the GPs and NPs is given in Box 4.2. What these findings illustrate is a number of key differences between the GPs and NPs when using information to make judgements and decisions. GPs articulated slightly fewer hypotheses than the NPs; NPs interpreted 50% more cues and evaluated more hypotheses than GPs. With the exception of one NP, all participants arrived at a

Scenario 4.3

Mrs James, a 70-year-old woman, presents at the surgery with a rash on her back and complaining of irritation at the site of the rash. How would you proceed?

Box 4.2 Summary of number of stages used by GPs and NPs in the decision making processes

Stages in the decision making processes	GPs (n = 11)	Mean per practitioner	% of GP	NPs (n = 11)	Mean per practitioner	% of NP
Cue acquisition	72	6.55	n/a	73	6.63	n/a
Hypothesis generation	7	0.64	n/a	12	1.09	n/a
Cue interpretation	2	0.21	n/a	4	0.36	n/a
Hypothesis evaluation	4	0.36	n/a	8	0.72	n/a
Correct diagnosis	11	n/a	100	10	n/a	91
Treatment:						
antiviral therapy	4	n/a	36	4	n/a	36
analgesics	7	n/a	64	1	n/a	9
symptoms only	2	n/a	18	1	n/a	9
antibiotics	2	n/a	18	1	n/a	9
Return to see NP/GP	4	n/a	36	5	n/a	45
Advice	8	n/a	73	6	n/a	54
Refer to GP				4	n/a	36
Time to complete scenario (min)	66	6.00	n/a	87	8.0	n/a

n/a, not applicable.

correct diagnosis of shingles. Antiviral therapy was the treatment choice for four GPs and NPs and a significantly higher proportion of GPs than NPs would prescribe analgesics. GPs were faster than NPs at completing the decision task(s) – 6 minutes as opposed to the NPs' 8 minutes.

All 11 GPs and 10 of the 11 NPs arrived at a correct diagnosis using three different ways of obtaining clinical information: focused questioning, patient examination and specific cues. A model answer identifying critical and relevant cues for a successful decision is outlined in Figure 4.1. Critical cues are those necessary for successful diagnosis of the condition and relevant cues are ones that provide important information for reaching an accurate diagnosis. Figure 4.2 provides a 'map' of the thought

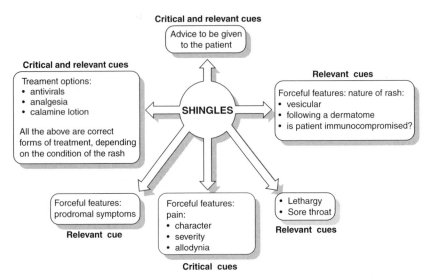

Figure 4.1 Critical and relevant cues for a successful decision.

processes used by the majority of GPs and NPs. The one NP who failed to correctly identify what was wrong with the patient failed to recognise the relevant information represented by the photograph. Consequently, her hypothesis evaluation and diagnosis were also incorrect.

What the results of this particular study and scenario indicate is that, overall, the decision making stages used by the two groups reveal a consistent pattern. When considering the use of both relevant and critical information, both groups focused on the critical cues evident in the photograph. This indicated that NPs and GPs selected similar important information to generate, organise and interpret data to reach their conclusion.

PRACTICAL TIPS FOR IMPROVING THE USE OF CUES

As has been illustrated, how nurses identify and use information is key to accurate judgement and decision making. The following suggestions are ways in which you can try to ensure that you use information effectively in your judgement and decision making (also see Ch. 5).

◆ *Case simulations* – can be used to test the discriminative abilities of nurses regarding the state of the patient and the weightings given to cues used in determining action or outcomes. Strategies utilised by

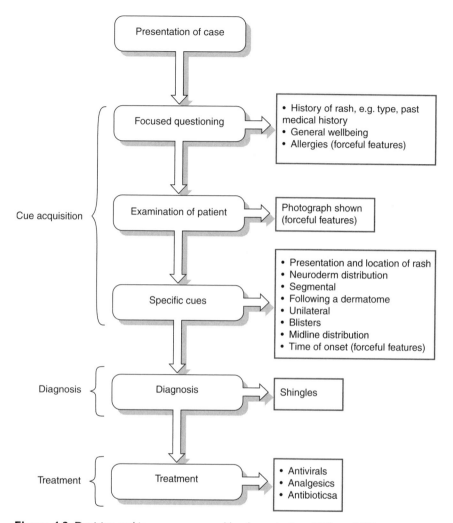

Figure 4.2 Decision making processes used by the majority of NPs and GPs.

nurses to make decisions can be identified and used to guide less experienced practitioners through the decision making process.

◆ *Ward-based teaching* – a more systematic approach to decision making, which emphasises reflexive, analytical skills and combines critical thinking with students' own practice could be adopted as part of staff development.

◆ *Integration of frequent decision making opportunities* – together with productive feedback, discussion and evaluation of both positive and negative consequences of decisions in daily practice on the ward.

◆ *Teaching strategies* – should help students by enabling them to understand the personal processes of thought so that they can analyse why a specific thought content arose or did not arise and what to do about it (Grant & Marsden, 1987).

◆ *Delay providing the actual diagnosis in teaching and simulations* – the resulting uncertainty allows critical clinical thinking to emerge (Grant & Marsden, 1987).

◆ *Encourage the use of probability estimates* – these help to foster clinical reasoning. Probability estimates are dependent on personal experiences and should be encouraged in both ward based and higher educational teaching so that nurses become accustomed to examining their decision making processes for possible biases developed from past experiences.

◆ *Develop a policy capturing framework* – this will provide feedback and awareness to nurses of the decisions and policies they have generated, is likely to be acceptable to them and should be encouraged as an aid to improving decision making (see Ch. 5).

CONCLUSION

The studies alluded to in this chapter have shown that, whilst nurse decision making may have a different focus from that of medicine, many of the processes used by doctors and nurses are more alike than some commentators would have us believe. Nurses should develop practice, educational and research responses that draw on the rich heritage of decision making research in areas such as medicine. There is no need for us to 'reinvent the wheel' in many cases. With the increasing focus on evidence based health care nurses need to be able to provide more articulate, logical and systematic reasons for their decisions. In this chapter, concrete and practical tips have been presented to help those practitioners who wish to take up these challenges.

QUESTIONS FOR DISCUSSION

◆ What systems are in place for evaluating the decisions offered to patients?

◆ Using patient scenarios (or a real patient) discuss with a colleague the steps taken for reaching your decisions and provide a rationale for them. Consider how much emphasis you attribute to each piece of clinical information and articulate your reasons.

◆ Consider how you could improve your own decision making processes.

ANNOTATED FURTHER READING

Russo, J. & Schoemaker, P.J.H. (1991). *Confident decision making.* London: Piatkus.

A good introduction to decision making. The book's informal style makes it easy to read. Although written with a commercial focus, some medical examples are included and these can easily be translated for nurse decision making.

Sutherland, S. (1992). *Irrationality: The enemy within.* London: Penguin.

This paperback presents an overview of the psychological processes relating to decision making. It looks at irrational behaviours and beliefs and provides an array of examples, including clinical ones. Some of the more serious discourses on decision making are dealt with in an explanatory manner, sometimes with a blend of humour.

Higgs, J. & Jones, M. (eds) (1995). *Clinical reasoning in the health professions.* Oxford: Butterworth-Heinemann.

This is a well structured and explanatory book on decision making in various health care professions and complements the others mentioned.

REFERENCES

Bryans, A. & McIntosh, J. (1996). Decision making in community nursing: An analysis of the stages of decision making as they relate to community nursing assessment practice. *Journal of Advanced Nursing, 24,* 24–36.

Cioffi, J. (2000). Nurses' experiences of making decisions to call emergency assistance to their patients. *Journal of Advanced Nursing, 32*(1), 108–114.

Elstein, A.S., Shulman, L.S., & Sprafka, S.A. (1978). *Medical problem solving: An analysis of clinical reasoning.* Cambridge, MA: Harvard.

Ericsson, K.A. & Simon, H.A. (1993). *Protocol analysis: Verbal reports as data.* Cambridge, MA: MIT Press.

Grant, J. & Marsden, P. (1987). The structure of memorized knowledge in students and clinicians: an explanation for diagnostic expertise. *Medical Education, 21,* 92–98.

Hallett, C., Austin, L., Caress, A., & Luker, K.A. (2000). Wound care in the community setting: Clinical decision making in context. *Journal of Advanced Nursing, 31*(4), 783–793.

Hammond, K.R. (1978). Toward increasing competence of thought in public policy formation. In Hammond, K.R. (ed.), *Judgement and decision in public policy formation* (pp. 11–32). Boulder, CO: Westview.

Hammond, K., Kelly, K., & Castellan, E.A. (1966). Clinical inference in nursing: Use of information seeking strategies by nurses. *Nursing Research, 15*(4), 330–336.

Lamond, D. (2000). The information content of the nurse change of shift report: A comparative study. *Journal of Advanced Nursing, 31*(4), 794–804.

Lamond, D.W., Crow, R., Chase, J., Doggen, K., & Swinkels, M. (1996). Information sources used in decision making: Considerations for simulation development. *International Journal of Nursing Studies, 33*(1), 47–57.

Luker, K.A. & Kenrick, M. (1992). An exploratory study of the sources of influence on the clinical decisions of community nurses. *Journal of Advanced Nursing, 17,* 437–446.

Marsden, J. (1999). Expert nurse decision making: Telephone triage in an ophthalmic accident and emergency department. *Nursing Times Research, 4*(1), 44–52.

Russo, J. & Schoemaker, P.J.H. (1991). *Confident decision making.* London: Piatkus.

Weinstein, M. & Fineberg, H. (1986). *Clinical Decision Analysis.* Philadelphia: W.B. Saunders.

White, J.E., Nativo, D.G., Kobert, S.N., & Engbert, S.J. (1992). Content and process in clinical decision making. *Journal of Nursing Scholarship, 24*(2), 153–158.

5

Interpretation of risk and social judgement theory

Dawn Dowding

KEY ISSUES

- Risk is unavoidable in clinical practice.
- Several ways of ascertaining risks in practice exist and can be used by nurses.
- Nurses should question the clinical usefulness of the tools commonly used to assess clinical risk.
- Social judgement theory offers a means of framing and managing risk in practice.

THE NATURE OF RISK IN CLINICAL PRACTICE

Individuals within society are no strangers to the concept of risk. We are aware of 'risks' on a variety of different levels: the risk of environmental pollution, the risk of being run over when we cross the road or the risk of developing lung cancer if we smoke.

The Royal Society (1992, p. 2) defines risk as 'the probability that a particular adverse event occurs during a stated period of time, or results from a particular challenge'. This definition has been criticised for defining risk too objectively (Heyman, 1998). In particular, it ignores the values individuals attach to different outcomes (not all of which we will all see negatively – such as disability) and the complexity of the social assessment of risk. Moreover, it focuses on single adverse events, rather than acknowledging the complex interaction of variables that occurs in real life. Another (less objective) definition of risk is 'the projection of a degree of uncertainty about the future on the external world' (Heyman, 1998, p. 5).

Although these definitions vary in the precision with which they define risk, they have two similarities: the inclusion of uncertainty or probability, and the process of prediction.

Uncertainty and health care are inseparable; health care practitioners operate in a world where outcomes cannot be predicted with certainty, for example, the exact probability or likelihood of a woman having a healthy baby. Instead, we try to quantify (or at least qualitatively categorise) the risks attached to that particular situation. For instance, based on the practitioners' expertise, the available research evidence and the woman's previous pregnancies, she may be considered to be a high risk case. The actual probability or likelihood of the negative event may not actually be known but is greater than those women considered as low risk. Although exact probabilities may not be known, we can see that these sorts of categorisations have some 'ordinal' properties.

Practitioners deal with risk all the time and from a variety of different perspectives. For instance, if you are a practice nurse screening your patients for coronary heart disease or cervical cancer, you are probably also involved in providing your patients with information about their risk of developing certain diseases. If you are a community psychiatric nurse, you may be involved in assessing the risk a client poses to the local community (in the form of 'how likely is it they will cause harm to someone else?'). If you work in an acute psychiatric environment, risk assessment may focus on the risk your client poses to themselves. If you work in a care of the elderly unit, assessing a patient's risk of developing pressure sores, or risk of falling, are common inputs into decision making. All of these judgements regarding risk are trying to predict what might happen. In other words, the nurses are attaching a certain probability to the event either happening or not happening. As Chapter 3 highlights, these types of judgement are integral to the practice of nursing and midwifery.

Clinical practice is often concerned with risk reduction and, with the upward trend in healthcare litigation, there is an increasing emphasis on risk management (for patients and staff). Managing risk involves trying to reduce the number of negative outcomes associated with an environment or procedure – all environments or procedures carry risks, to a greater or lesser extent. One may assess a patient as at risk of developing pressure sores, or falling out of bed, and then implement measures to try to reduce the likelihood of this event occurring (e.g. via specialist mattresses or cot sides). In mental health, an individual may be assessed as being at risk of harming themselves, leading to interventions designed to reduce this risk to themselves, such as being observed continuously by a member of staff.

When considering risk assessment and risk reduction, it is vital that the initial assessment of risk is accurate. The potential financial cost of implementing procedures to reduce risk unnecessarily is enormous. For instance, if one were to erroneously assess all patients in a nursing home as at risk of developing pressure sores and provide all of them with (expensive) therapeutic mattresses, the costs of care would soon spiral out of control. However, the implications of not correctly identifying an individual at risk of developing a pressure sore may also exert significant costs: increased nursing care to heal the sore, greater potential for complaints regarding the quality of care received and the costs of drugs or medical devices.

Risk, then, is integral to nursing and midwifery practice and the assessment of risk is one of the most common judgements nurses, midwives and health visitors make.

ASSESSING RISK

One of the ways in which judgements of risk have been formalised is through the use of risk assessment tools or diagnostic tests. For instance, the well established instruments for assessing an individual's risk of developing coronary heart disease based on data from the Framingham heart study (Isles et al., 2000). Similarly, most nurses working in acute or long term care will be familiar with the use of pressure sore risk assessment tools, such as the Braden or Waterlow scales. In psychiatric care a number of risk assessment tools exist to try and establish an individual's risk of harming themselves or being violent (Holdsworth et al., 1999). Most of these tools collect data regarding various factors thought to be associated with the event of interest (be it a myocardial infarction, a violent event or the development of pressure sores). There is normally some form of scoring system, so the higher (or lower) a score the individual receives the higher (or lower) the probability of the event occurring.

To reduce risk it is often necessary to distinguish at risk cases from not at risk cases. This is often done by generating some form of cut off point. For example, the Braden scale uses the cut off point of 17 or below to define individuals considered at risk of developing pressure sores (VandenBosch et al., 1996).

The key issues when examining risk assessment tools is how good are they at distinguishing those at risk from those who are not; and are they better or more accurate than simply relying on professional judgement. To explore the issues in some detail, examples will be used from coronary heart disease screening and pressure sore risk assessment. However, the concepts applied in this part of the chapter are equally applicable to any form of assessment tool.

The main criterion against which risk assessment tools, screening instruments or other forms of diagnostic test are evaluated is their ability to correctly identify individuals likely to develop the disease or condition (true positives) and individuals unlikely to develop the disease or condition (true negatives). Most of the tests used in health care are not 100% accurate and so will always identify some individuals as being at high risk when (in truth) they are not – false positives. Or, conversely, they will identify some individuals as being at low risk when, in reality, they are not (false negatives). A good risk assessment tool minimises the number of false positives and false negatives it identifies. The formal terms for a tool's accuracy are sensitivity (its ability to identify true positive cases) and specificity (its ability to identify true negative cases).

Table 5.1 shows the sensitivity and specificity results for three types of coronary heart disease risk assessment tool (taken from Wallis et al., 2000) and for the Braden scale, which measures pressure sore risk (taken from VandenBosch et al., 1996). What you, as a practitioner, need to know is how to use this information in clinical practice.

Imagine you are a nurse practitioner running a screening clinic for over 65s in your local health centre. You have just interviewed Mr Smith and carried out an assessment for his risk of developing coronary heart disease over the next 10 years. The Joint British chart, suggests he has a > 20% risk.

Table 5.1 Sensitivity and specificity of coronary heart disease screening tools and the Braden scale (VandenBosch et al., 1996; Wallis et al., 2000)

Coronary risk screening tool	15% risk of heart disease over 10 years		20% risk of heart disease over 10 years	
	Sensitivity (%)	Specificity (%)	Sensitivity (%)	Specificity (%)
Sheffield table	98	91	81	96
Joint British chart	91	98	63	98
New Zealand chart	93	89	75	96
Braden scale	59	59		

Table 5.2 Sensitivity and specificity – the Braden scale

Prevalence of pressure sores in population (%)	Identified 'at risk' Sensitivity 59%		Identified 'not at risk' Specificity 59%		Predictive value of being 'at risk' (positive test) (%)	Predictive value of being 'not at risk' (negative test) (%)
	Actually at risk	Incorrectly identified	Actually not at risk	Incorrectly identified		
5	3	39	56	2	7.1	96.5
20	12	33	47	8	26.7	85.5

However, this particular chart has a sensitivity of 63%, and a specificity of 98%. This means that although identified as high risk, the chart picks up only 63% of such cases accurately (meaning that there is a 37% chance of telling him he is at high risk when in reality he is not). However, because the chart has a high specificity, of 98%, if he had been identified as a low risk, you could probably be fairly happy that this was a reasonably accurate result (there is only a 2% chance that he will be a false negative or actually at risk).

However, interpretations of results like this are not as simple as just looking at the sensitivity and specificity of test results. As we saw in Chapter 2, the base rate or prevalence of a condition is also important when looking at the accuracy of assessment tool results. As an example, look at Table 5.2, relating to the Braden scale (VandenBosch et al., 1996).

The table might look daunting at first, but if you work through the numbers systematically its importance will become clear. If you assume that the risk assessment tool has been used on 100 people, with the baseline prevalence of pressure sores being 5%, this means five people out of the

100 will develop sores. The tool has a specificity of 59%, so it will accurately identify 59% of these, or three people; the other two will be mistakenly categorised as being at low risk. The tool also has a specificity of 59%, so it will accurately identify 59% of the 95 who are not at risk of developing sores, or 56 of them; the remaining 39 will be inaccurately identified as being at risk of developing sores when they are not. This means that, because the prevalence of sores is so low, only three individuals, out of the 42 identified as being at risk, or 7% of them, will actually be at risk. This is the predictive value of the assessment tool, for high risk cases. As you can see from Table 5.2, if the prevalence of pressure sores in your population is 20% (higher than before), then the number of individuals actually at risk increases, so the predictive value of the assessment tool also increases, this time to 26%.

So, if you are using some form of assessment tool, screening tool, or diagnostic tool in practice, you need to know:

◆ how good is it at identifying high risk or positive cases
◆ how good is it at identifying low risk or negative cases
◆ the prevalence of the condition it is assessing in the general population.

If you have all of this information, you can decide what the tool is actually telling you about the person's risk of developing the disease or condition. These principles are just as relevant when considering whether someone is a suicide risk, when counselling a mother on the results of a fetal abnormality screening test or when assessing the risk of developing other types of disease.

Also, as already mentioned, you need to be aware of how good the risk assessment tool is in comparison to professional judgements of risk alone. Ideally, you would like to be using a risk assessment tool that is more accurate than professional judgement exercised in isolation – otherwise there is no need to use the tool at all. An example of this is highlighted by VandenBosch et al. (1996). They compared the predictive validity of the Braden Score with nurses' judgements of pressure sore risk for a total of 103 patients. They found that nurses' sensitivity was 51.7% and their specificity 58.9%, compared to the results for the Braden scale (which were displayed in Table 5.2 on page 85). The Braden scale has a sensitivity of 59% and a specificity of 59% (when the cut off point is 17). So the scale was only slightly better than professional judgement when identifying 'at risk' cases, and the same as professional judgement for identifying 'not at risk' cases. In this instance, one has to question the usefulness of the risk assessment tool.

ANALYSING RISK THROUGH SOCIAL JUDGEMENT THEORY

Thus far the chapter has highlighted how judgements regarding risk are part of a broader range of judgements that nurses and midwives make in their clinical practice. Chapter 2 illustrated that inaccuracy and variation can have a significant effect on the care that patients receive. Examining judgement and decision making in health care, and the information used to help 'feed' these processes, is vital. One way of examining information use between individuals is social judgement theory, which builds on the theoretical work of Brunswik, who is responsible for the lens model on which the theory is based (Fig. 5.1). The model's left hand side represents the ecological or real situation, that is, what is really wrong with the patient. A variety of different information cues are directly linked to this real situation (such as patient signs and symptoms). Each of these cues has different weights attached to it. Clinicians use these cues to make their judgement, which is represented on the right hand side of the model. How good an individual clinician's judgement is can be ascertained by

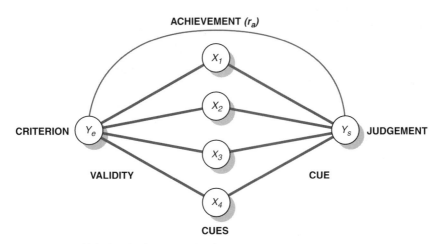

- Y_e is the criterion or actual patient state
- X_1–X_n are the cues that are related to the patient state. They may vary in importance, or 'weight', with regard to their relationship to the patient state
- Y_s is the person's judgement about the criterion or patient state. The person can use the cues X_n in a different way to how they are actually related to Y_e
- r_a is the person's achievement

Figure 5.1 Brunswik's lens model. Reproduced with permission from Hammond et al. (1975, p. 274).

how the information cues have been used. If they are weighted in ways that mirror the association with the ecological situation then the judgement will be accurate. However, if the individual weights the importance of cues differently, then the judgement will not reflect the ecological situation (Cooksey, 1996).

Statistical multiple regression techniques are used to model how information cues relate to the patient state and individual judgement. These models represent the way information is linked to the 'real' patient state and allow comparison between clinicians, equations and policies. The recommended reading at the end of the chapter provides more detailed starting points for exploring the statistics behind the technique, here, we will focus on how to apply the techniques in practice.

APPLYING SOCIAL JUDGEMENT THEORY TO PRACTICE

To illustrate how the principles of social judgement theory may be applied to clinical practice, consider Scenario 5.1.

Scenario 5.1

You are a staff nurse in charge of an acute psychiatric unit. A 20-year-old male is admitted to your ward after trying to jump off a bridge into the local river. He has refused to give his name or address to the police officers who have accompanied him to the hospital and he doesn't have any identification on him. However, when he appears on your ward one of your students is adamant that they have looked after him before, when on placement in another ward within your institution. The man doesn't seem to be depressed, he isn't vocalising any suicidal thoughts and, when talking to you on admission, appears perfectly logical and pleasant. However, he will not discuss what he was doing on the bridge. His clothes are expensive and he appears to care for himself well. The student tells you that if it is the same man, he has a history of suicidal intent and has been admitted to several psychiatric units after similar incidents.

The social judgement model suggests the man's actual state (whether or not he may harm himself for instance) is linked to a number of cues present within the environment. For instance, his age, gender, previous medical history and current behaviour. As a clinician, you need to make a judgement about his actual state (whether he is at risk of harming himself) using the information available to you – his age, previous medical history and current behaviour. You may feel that certain bits of information are more important than others when making this judgement, for instance his unwillingness to explain to you what he was doing on the bridge may influence your judgement considerably. How 'good' your judgement is will depend on how well your use of the information (and the importance you attach to it) matches the 'real' situation. For instance, your student might indeed have cared for the man previously and the information regarding his previous history is vital for an accurate judgement. However, you might choose to ignore the information the student gives you because you feel that it is not likely to be accurate. You therefore judge incorrectly that he is unlikely to harm himself, and make decisions for treatment based on this.

The social judgement model can also explain how two different judges reach different judgements using exactly the same information (Fig. 5.2): different judges weigh the importance of information cues differently, naturally leading to different judgements. For instance, using the previous example, supposing another staff nurse commences a shift in the afternoon and the student again explains the man's previous history. You ignored this information, but the new staff nurse feels it is highly important, weights it as such in the judgement forming process, and concludes that the man is at high risk of harming himself – the direct opposite of your opinion. The basis of this discrepancy is the different information you both used to inform your judgement, together with the differing levels of importance you attached to information.

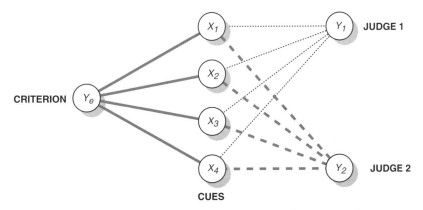

Figure 5.2 Lens model illustrating how two judges can reach different judgements. Reproduced from Cooksey (1996, p. 68).

The above situation shows how social judgement theory can explain or describe why errors in judgement can occur in clinical practice. This is important when trying to investigate how judgements (and subsequent treatment) can vary in clinical practice. Social judgement approaches can also be used to improve clinical practice. For instance, suppose you became extremely bothered by the lack of accuracy of your judgements and the variability in the judgements of the staff on your unit. One of the strategies that could be used would be to try and capture the 'real world' (or ecological situation) in some form of statistical equation, which you could use when making similar judgements in the future – this is sometimes known as policy capturing.

For instance, using the previous scenario, the social judgement approach suggests that certain information cues will be correlated with the risk of the man committing suicide. Firstly, you could try to identify the left hand side of the lens model and capture how different clinical cues predict suicide risk. This could be achieved by examining the notes and charts of all the patients in your clinical area over a period of time and extracting all the relevant information cues, together with checking the relevant literature. This would give you a list of possible information cues that predict suicide risk. Using multiple regression techniques you could examine how these cues are related to the risk of suicide (or parasuicide). This would give you an equation, indicating the information needed to make a prediction and the relative importance of different types of information.

Once armed with this information, you could then compare how your nurses make judgements about suicide risk compared to the 'real' situation. You might find that actually their judgements are not too bad! However, the likelihood is that they will use information inconsistently to make judgements. You could help them to improve their accuracy by showing them how their judgement policies (equations) match the real situation, and giving them feedback on how to alter the information they use to make judgements so that weighting and cue use is more consistent. Alternatively, you might decide to try and use your risk assessment equation in the form of an assessment tool or computerised decision support tool.

Examples of the use of such judgement policy techniques are more prevalent in medicine than in nursing. However, exceptions do exist. For example, Rosenthal et al. (1992) examined how nurse practitioners made diagnostic judgements regarding chlamydial infection. They examined the judgement policies of nurses in practice and compared them to an algorithm based on the real situation. Using an algorithm reduced the inconsistency with which cues are used and ensured only relevant information for the judgement was used. The findings of this study mirror those in medicine (e.g. de Dombal, 1988; Goldman et al., 1988; Skånér et al., 1998; Westenberg et al., 1998). Analysis of judgement processes using lens model techniques have shown that human judges use information inconsistently, often weighting irrelevant information for the judgement task as important. Moreover, using statistical equations – or computer protocols based on these equations – can reduce inconsistency and improve judgement.

WHY USE SOCIAL JUDGEMENT APPROACHES?

As has been highlighted in the previous sections in this chapter, risk assessment is one of a number of judgements nurses, midwives and health visitors make in clinical practice. To ensure that patients and clients receive the best quality care wherever they are treated, regardless of who is caring for them, it is imperative that *how* practitioners make judgements impacting on care is examined systematically. The approach advocated by social judgement theorists allows for the examination of the accuracy of judgements. Moroever, it also captures the accuracy of instruments designed to enhance professional judgements such as pressure sore or suicide risk assessment tools. Social judgement theory is also a normative theory; the approach suggests ways in which judgements can be improved and presents solutions via the relatively transparent mode of statistical modelling.

It is important to acknowledge that there are limitations attached to the use of social judgement theory. Specifically, the approach:

◆ assumes the information attached to a judgement situation in the environment can be identified
◆ assumes that information is linked to a particular situation in a consistent fashion (for example, patients who are very thin and immobile will always be at high risk of pressure sore development, despite other factors)
◆ often uses vignettes (rather than 'real' patient cases) to examine how practitioners make judgements (and actual behaviour in practice might be very different to that identified in research studies).

This last point, however, is not as troublesome as it might at first seem. Examination of practice using vignettes can provide a safe environment within which to examine judgement variation. In the long term, the vignette and social judgement combination could provide a useful educational tool to ensure that judgements are more consistent in practice.

CONCLUSION

The intention of this chapter was to encourage you to consider the processes of risk assessment and associated judgements in more detail. It is not advocating that you should use social judgement theory to analyse every clinical situation that you encounter. Rather, we hope that it has made you aware of some of the important issues when carrying out risk assessment judgements or using assessment/screening tools. So next time you make a judgement in your practice area, or use some form of risk assessment tool, consider the following:

◆ What information have you used to make that judgement?
◆ What weighting or importance have you attached to certain types of information? Is there one piece of information in particular that you have used which is the basis of your judgement?
◆ What evidence do you have that the information you have used is relevant to the judgement situation?
◆ How accurate is your judgement? Have you considered what the base rate, or prevalence, is of the condition/situation within the patient group you are working with? Could there be another explanation?

If you are using risk assessment tools to support your decisions:

◆ What research evidence are they based on?
◆ Do you have evidence to suggest that they are any better than using your own judgement?

In summary, thinking about risk and the judgements you make in clinical practice is important for patient care. As highlighted in previous chapters, judgements are the foundations of decision making in health care. If your judgement is inaccurate, then the decisions taken on the basis of that judgement will most likely be wrong in some regard. For instance, if you judge (inaccurately) that a patient is at high risk of developing sores, then act appropriately (by providing a therapeutic mattress, for instance). The patient will have received appropriate treatment, albeit based on inaccurate judgement. In this case, it is not particularly serious. However, consider the potential consequences of inaccurately judging a woman as a low risk case during her pregnancy and treating her as such? Appropriate treatment based on inaccurate judgement suddenly takes on a far more serious face.

ANNOTATED FURTHER READING

For those interested in reading further about social judgement theory/analysis, the following texts are useful (however, they do cover the area in some complexity).

Cooksey, R.W. (1996). *Judgment analysis: Theory, methods and applications.* San Diego: Academic Press.

Katz, M.F. & Schwartz, S. (1975). *Human judgement and decision processes.* New York: Academic Press. (In particular, the chapter by Hammond et al. on social judgement theory.)

REFERENCES

Cooksey, R.W. (1996). *Judgment analysis: Theory, methods and applications.* San Diego: Academic Press.

de Dombal, F.T. (1988). Computer-aided diagnosis of acute abdominal pain: The British experience. In: Dowie, J. & Elstein, A. (eds), *Professional judgment. A reader in clinical decision making* (pp. 190–199). Cambridge: Cambridge University Press.

Goldman, L., Cook, E.F., Brand, D.A. et al. (1988). A computer protocol to predict myocardial infarction in emergency department patients with chest pain. *New England Journal of Medicine, 318*(13), 797–803.

Hammond, K.R., Stewart, T.R., Brehmer, B., & Steinmann, D.O. (1975). Social judgment theory. In: Katz, M.F. & Schwartz, S. (eds), *Human judgment and decision processes* (pp. 271–312). New York: Academic Press.

Heyman, B. (1998). Introduction. In: Heyman, B. (ed.), *Risk, health and health care. A qualitative approach* (pp. 1–23). London: Arnold.

Holdsworth, N., Collis, B., & Allott, R. (1999). The development and evaluation of a brief risk screening instrument for the psychiatric inpatient setting. *Journal of Psychiatric and Mental Health Nursing, 6,* 43–52.

Isles, C.G., Ritchie, L.D., Murchie, P., & Norrie, J. (2000). Risk assessment in primary prevention of coronary heart disease: randomised comparison of three scoring methods. *British Medical Journal, 320,* 690–691.

Rosenthal, G.E., Mettler, G., Pare, S., Riegger, M., Ward, M., & Landefeld, C.S. (1992). Diagnostic judgements of nurse practitioners providing primary gynecologic care: A quantitative analysis. *Journal of General Internal Medicine, 7,* 304–311.

Royal Society (1992) *Risk: Analysis, perception and management. Report of a Royal Society study group.* London: The Royal Society.

Skånér, Y., Strender, L.E., & Bring, J. (1998). How do GPs use clinical information in their judgements of heart failure? A clinical judgement analysis study. *Scandinavian Journal of Primary Health Care, 16,* 95–100.

VandenBosch, T., Montoye, C., Satwicz, M., Durkee-Leonard, K., & Boylan-Lewis, B. (1996). Predictive validity of the Braden scale and nurse perception in identifying pressure ulcer risk. *Applied Nursing Research, 9*(2), 80–86.

Wallis, E.J., Ramsay, L.E., Yikona, J.I.N.M., & Jackson, P.R. (2000). Comparison of methods of estimating coronary risk. *British Medical Journal, 321,* 17.

Westenberg, M.R.M., Koele, P., & Kools, E. (1998). The treatment of substance addicts: A judgement analysis of therapists' matching strategies. *Clinical Psychology and Psychotherapy, 5,* 39–46.

6

What decisions do nurses make?

Dorothy McCaughan

KEY ISSUES

◆ Nurses make a limited number of types of clinical decisions (even though the focus of clinical decisions is wide ranging).

◆ Many nursing decisions are amenable to the application of the findings of healthcare research.

◆ We need to know about decisions nurses make as a key stage in the development of an evidence base for nursing.

◆ Human sources of information are the most powerful force in influencing real life clinical decision making.

WHY DO WE NEED TO KNOW ABOUT THE DECISIONS THAT NURSES MAKE?

A large proportion of the research literature on nurse decision making focuses on the processes of decision making, rather than on the nature of the decisions that nurses make. Nurses form the largest professional group working within the NHS, yet we know surprisingly little about the kinds of decisions they make in their routine, day to day, clinical practice. As traditional professional boundaries between doctors and nurses, and nurses and support workers, become increasingly blurred and, as new and expanded roles in nursing develop, it would seem the time is ripe for a detailed examination of the kinds of decisions nurses are currently making in practice.

Today, in most clinical settings, members of a multidisciplinary team work together to provide what they hope is optimal patient care. Many different professionals can contribute to a single decision, or a series of decisions, taken on behalf of a patient (think of discharge planning for a patient who has suffered a stroke), and it can be difficult to disentangle the specific contribution of the nurse to this complex and sometimes protracted decision making process. Yet it is essential for nurse education and training that we recognise and understand the nurse's contribution to this kind of shared decision making activity.

Also, with the increasing emphasis on the need for all health care professionals to use 'evidence' to inform their practice, there is a need to look at the ways in which nurses routinely incorporate information into their decision making. It is only when the types of decisions that nurses make have been identified, along with the sources of information (research based or otherwise) that they currently use, that consideration can be given to how amenable their decisions are to the application of research evidence. If research evidence is to be incorporated routinely into practice, it must provide answers to the questions that clinicians ask routinely. There is a large and growing body of research showing that nurses do not routinely utilise research findings in practice, and the reasons why they reject them have been well documented in both the US (Funk et al., 1995) and the UK (Dunn et al., 1998). If researchers are to reach practitioners with their messages for practice, they need to know about those sources of information that nurses actually use when faced with clinical challenges incorporating decision choices, and they need an explanation of why these sources have been chosen.

To effectively serve practitioners making decisions affecting patient care, researchers need to know:

◆ the kinds of decisions nurses make
◆ the information that nurses require to help them make these decisions
◆ how to present good quality (i.e. research based) information to nurses in ways that are most acceptable to practitioners.

Therefore, knowledge of the kinds of decisions nurses make in practice is a prerequisite for the development of an evidence base that will match their needs for information. The rest of this chapter considers the issue of what decisions nurses make in practice in more detail.

WHAT DECISIONS DO NURSES ACTUALLY MAKE?

Clinical decision making is an intrinsic part of clinical practice and clinical decisions necessarily involve choices between discrete options. To attempt to answer the question 'what decisions do nurses actually make?' I will draw on the findings of an NHS Research & Development (NHS R&D) study, which investigated nurses' use of research information in clinical decision making in acute (medical and surgical) hospital wards and coronary care units (Thompson et al., 2000). The following discussion is therefore specific to the areas of acute medical, surgical and coronary care. However, some of the types of decisions identified are equally applicable to nurses and midwives practising in a variety of different health care environments.

The project employed a case study approach with multiple methods of data collection to examine how nurses use research information in their clinical decisions. Purposive sampling led to in-depth interviews ($n = 108$) being conducted with nurses with a wide range of professional and educational qualifications, including a number of clinical nurse special-ists. The interviews were supplemented by periods of observation of the same nurses going about their daily duties (periods of 2–3 hours observa-tion; 180 hours in total). A prime consideration in the design of the study was that it should seek to describe the types of decisions that nurses *actu-ally* make in their day to day practice, as opposed to those decisions that nurses *say* they make. Observation was therefore the method of choice to explore decision making as it occurred in 'real time', in the context of the busy clinical environment with all its time constraints, pressures of work prioritisation and continual interruptions and distractions. During data collection, the observer enacted the role of 'observer as participant', asking the nurse to clarify aspects of his or her decision making where necessary.

Further information on the decisions made was generated via a Q methodological modelling exercise. Q methodology is a technique used for the statistical modelling of shared views and values. Contrasting locations (different clinical environments) were selected to try to discern any effect exerted by clinical specialty on decision making behaviour (Crow et al.,1995).

The focus of decisions

The decisions reported by nurses during interviews, and those that they were observed to make in the ward or unit, are presented in Box 6.1.

The areas of nursing activity identified in this study do not differ greatly from those described elsewhere (Benner, 1984; Carr-Hill et al., 1992; Jinks & Hope, 2000). It is the detailed description of the types of decisions taken by nurses that is newly reported in this study. The majority of decisions actually made by nurses could be included in a six-fold taxonomy of decision types (Table 6.1) and the largest number of decisions was related to questions of treatment or intervention. This is to say that, decisions were primarily concerned with questions of clinical effectiveness. As such, they could easily be translated into focused clinical questions, eminently amenable to the evidence based approach of searching and appraising the research literature, and implementing change where appropriate, as described in Chapter 7.

Frequency of decision making

Interview data revealed that nurses found it difficult to describe the kinds of decisions they took on a daily basis in abstract terms. However, they responded well to a question asking them mentally to 'run through' the

Box 6.1 The focus of decisions in acute care areas

◆ Dressings.

◆ Pressure sore monitoring/prevention/use of devices.

◆ Checking/monitoring observations/fluid intake/output.

◆ Patient hygiene.

◆ Patient mobility.

◆ Patient positioning.

◆ Infection control.

◆ Nutrition.

◆ Intravenous/oral fluids.

◆ Timing of premedications (in conjunction with theatre staff).

◆ Patient compliance, for example, medication.

◆ Referral to colleague/senior nurse/doctors/clinical nurse specialists/therapists/pharmacist.

◆ Referral to relatives/involvement of relatives, especially at times of patient admission and discharge.

◆ Interpreting results, mainly of blood tests and exercise tolerance tests.

◆ Decision to document care given.

◆ Bed management.

◆ Staffing/skill mix/allocation of patients to teams/delegation to juniors.

◆ General administration of ward, for example, checking drug stock levels.

◆ Staff development.

◆ Supervision/training of staff.

decisions they had taken during a previous shift in relation to the specific tasks they had carried out. The majority of nurses (although not the clinical nurse specialists) stressed the short amount of time they had available to make decisions generally and they described shifts where they needed to respond to decision situations with a series of 'quick fire' choices. One period of observation (lasting approximately 3 hours) disclosed a 'decision list' of 18 decisions, an average of one decision for every 10 minutes on duty.

The decisions taken over the course of a few hours by one E grade staff nurse on a medical ward are presented in Box 6.2.

Watson (1994) found an even more intense volume of decision making in a small study of nurses (*n* = 11) in the acute medical/surgical context, where observation over a 2 hour period revealed 18 decisions made.

Table 6.1 Decision types and associated clinical questions (Thompson et al., 2000)

Decision type	Exemplar decision	Exemplar question
Intervention/effectiveness: this type of decision involves choosing between interventions	Choosing a mattress for a frail elderly man who has been admitted with an acute bowel obstruction	In elderly and inactive patients, who may require surgical intervention, which is the most suitable pressure relieving mattress to prevent pressure sores?
Targeting: this is, strictly speaking, a subcategory of the intervention/effectiveness decisions outlined above. These decisions are of the form, 'choosing which patient will most benefit from the intervention'	Deciding which patients should get anti-embolic stockings	Is there a risk assessment tool available that will accurately predict which group of patients will benefit most from anti-embolic stockings?
Timing: again, a subcategory of intervention/effectiveness decisions. These commonly take the form of choosing the best time to deploy the intervention	Choosing a time to commence asthma education with newly diagnosed asthmatics	When to commence asthma education with newly diagnosed asthmatics?
Communication: this type of decision commonly focuses on choices relating to ways of delivering and receiving information to and from patients, families or colleagues. Sometimes these decisions are specifically related to the communication of risks and benefits of different interventions or prognostic categories	Choosing how to approach cardiac rehabilitation following acute myocardial infarction in an elderly patient who lives alone, although their family is nearby	Would I be better talking and explaining rehab with the patient's family present so that a clear understanding is obtained prior to the patient's discharge?
Service organisation, delivery and management: this type of decision concerns the configuration or processes of service delivery	Choosing how to organise handover so that communication is most effective	How should I organise handover so that the most effective form of communicating information results?
Experiential, understanding or hermeneutic: this relates to the interpretation of cues in the process of care	Choosing how to reassure a patient who is worrying about cardiac arrest after witnessing another patient arresting	How best do you reassure a patient who has witnessed someone having a cardiac arrest?

Box 6.2 The observed decisions of one acute medical ward staff nurse in a 3 hour period

◆ Decides to allow a dressing to stay in place on a woman with a large sacral pressure sore.

◆ Decides that a patient can be discharged if her blood results are normal.

◆ Shared decision with the bed coordinator regarding bed management.

◆ Decides to check that a patient has signed a consent form.

◆ Decides to move a patient into a side room after chemotherapy.

◆ Decides to ring the dietician for advice regarding the management of a diabetic patient and how best to manage a patient previously treated with total parenteral nutrition and who is now not eating.

◆ Decides what information to impart to patients' relatives regarding their conditions.

◆ Decides on the appropriateness of meals for the numerous diabetic patients at lunchtime.

◆ Decides on the optimal balance of skills during staff lunch breaks for staff.

◆ Decides to call the doctor regarding whether or not a patient can have aspirin.

◆ Decides to refer a patient to the palliative care clinical nurse specialist.

◆ Decides to place a patient on a pressure relieving mattress.

◆ Decides to give (prescribed) analgesia as a response to patient request.

◆ Decides to refer a patient with niggling chest pain to the doctor.

◆ Decides what advice to give a colleague who asks for advice regarding the taking of a wound swab.

◆ Decides to refer a patient with a sore mouth to the clinical nurse specialist.

◆ Decides that a patient who was to be discharged should now not be because the patient doesn't fully understand her self-medication programme.

◆ Decides to phone the colonoscopy clinic for advice regarding the diet of a patient going for endoscopy.

Bucknall (2000), in a study of 18 nurses in urban and rural based critical care settings, recorded an average of frequency of decision activities during 2 hours of observation of 238. If this figure is divided by the number of minutes observed, it was calculated that a patient care decision was made approximately every 30 seconds.

In our own study, observation of clinical nurse specialists suggested that, for this group of nurses at least, decision making could sometimes be a more leisurely process, allowing the decision maker time to plan ahead (including accessing and using research materials) or (as was revealed in interviews with nurses) time to reflect on a decision after the event and store the experience for future reference. Nurses working on medical and surgical wards mentioned reflection as an activity most frequently associated with decisions that had 'gone wrong' in some way, for example, drug errors or mistakes in the administration of blood transfusions.

The collaborative nature of decision making

Decision making in its clinical context was found to be a social activity usually involving more than one clinician, mirroring the findings of Cioffi (2000) and others. Nurses rarely took decisions alone, on any aspect of care, and constantly sought 'information' in the form of advice from their colleagues and other professionals on how to act when faced with uncertainty. The people selected (doctors, pharmacists, senior nurses or clinical nurse specialists) were perceived to have information particularly appropriate to that clinical situation, revealing that individual nurses drew on collective knowledge and experience whenever they gauged their own to be inadequate for the decision that faced them. In so far as decision making occurred as a shared activity, the nurses' decisions were shaped and moulded through the contributions of others, undergoing refinement as each new piece of information was accumulated. As well as gathering information from colleagues, nurses frequently sought confirmation from them that they were making the 'right' decision; thereby, perhaps subconsciously, spreading responsibility for any repercussions resulting from the decision taken.

When decisions were not taken

Observation on the wards revealed instances when an individual nurse, or a group of nurses, failed to recognise a potential decision making task; an omission that could have serious repercussions for the patient(s) involved. One striking example of this was observed when an elderly patient on a medical ward was 'allowed' to develop a pressure sore over a number of days because no one took the initial decision to begin preventive measures.

At times, observation showed procrastination and transference to be common features of both individual and collective nurse decision making, expressed through the use of terms such as 'let's wait and see' or 'we'll need to keep an eye on that'. The frequent outcome of such a period of 'watchful waiting' was that individual nurses were disinclined to make a choice personally and would refer to another member of staff (e.g. doctor or clinical nurse specialist) in the expectation of that person making a decision. This was a whole different category of decision making in itself: the decision to get someone else to make a decision.

Preferred sources of information to aid decision making

As indicated above, human sources of information were overwhelmingly preferred to text sources, with the exception of the *British National Formulary*, which was referred to frequently. Guidelines and protocols were used on only four occasions during 180 hours of observation, although there were many examples of 'missed opportunities' for using them, when nurses were clearly uncertain how to act and would have benefited from referring to them. For instance, on one occasion a newly qualified nurse was observed assisting an inexperienced house doctor to insert a fine bore feeding tube in a patient who had suffered a stroke. Neither of them had carried out the procedure before, although they had both seen it being performed. The doctor asked several questions of the nurse, who was unable to provide answers ('What size of tube do we need to use?', 'Can we put his medicines down the tube?', 'Do I need to use lubricating gel to insert the tube?'). The nurse could have accessed a protocol for the insertion of the tube from a file located in the office (found during a recent audit of documentation) only a few feet away from the procedure, but either was unaware of its existence or chose not to use it.

Another source that the majority of nurses interviewed described as playing a large part in their decision making was their own 'intuition', particularly those who were experienced in working in one clinical specialty over a long period of time. This mirrors the large amount of existing research showing that nurses rely on intuitive judgements in clinical situations (Pyles & Stern, 1983; Schrader & Fischer, 1987; Young, 1987). The nurses defined intuitive feelings as a 'gut reaction', 'a hunch that something is wrong', 'he just had a look about him', and would pursue their instinct to act even though clinical observations (blood pressure or pulse readings) might indicate that the patient had not deteriorated. Those nurses working in coronary care ascribed their intuitive feelings to their detailed knowledge of one specific group of clients and they drew on their personal 'memory bank' of past patients to help them decide how to act.

One interviewee, a registered nurse in one of the coronary care units, described intuition as follows:

I don't know ... some people would have no outward signs of anything. Their observations would be fine, their blood pressure would be fine, their heart rate would be fine. And you'll just look, and you'll think, you're not well. I've got an awful feeling you're not going to make it. And I remember one night I was on, and these relatives wanted to go home, and I remember saying to them, I don't think you should. If it was my mum, I certainly wouldn't want to go home. And I do know that you care a lot and want to be with her. And they said, well, the doctor said she's fine. And I said, well there's nothing I can put my finger on, but I don't think she's as well as she looks. So he said, are you telling me my mum's going to die? And I said to them, well I hope not, but there is that chance. And I certainly wouldn't ... I'm not happy for you to go home. And she arrested and died a couple of hours later. And I think possibly if I hadn't been around and seen a lot, then I know some say it's intuition, but I think you need to have been around and seen things to have that intuition really.

Cioffi (2000) and Benner and Tanner (1987) highlight the importance of the relationship between experience and the ability to make complex decisions in nursing practice. Their arguments indicate the importance of experience in the development of clinical decision making skills.

WHAT DIFFERENCE DOES KNOWING THESE DECISIONS MAKE FOR PRACTICE AND RESEARCH?

A focus on the kinds of decisions that nurses are making in the clinical context provides clarification about the scope of nursing practice at a time when nursing roles are fast evolving and nurses are taking on new roles and responsibilities. If nurses are to practise as autonomous and accountable practitioners, taking responsibility for the decisions they make, they need to be able to define what these decisions are and provide a rationale for how they make them.

Knowledge of the clinical decisions that nurses make should enable researchers to focus on those areas of nursing care of primary relevance to practitioners. It should enable them to respond to the needs of clinicians by providing systematic reviews of evidence where such evidence exists. Where such evidence does not exist, primary research can be targeted towards those areas where there is a clear need for evidence. A greater awareness of the decisions that clinicians face on a daily basis in practice should also assist the research community in prioritising which questions need to be answered first.

It is necessary to know about the decisions nurses make and the information sources they use to develop strategies designed to improve decision outcomes. The findings of our own study (Thompson et al., 2000) have shown that the passive dissemination of guidelines to practitioners does not work because they are not accessed at the time that decisions are actually being made. These findings are similar to those of others. For instance, Thomas and colleagues (1999) in a systematic review of clinical guidelines in nursing, midwifery and the therapies, suggest that active dissemination strategies can be more effective than passive dissemination in bringing about change. The authors of *Getting evidence into practice* (Effective Health Care Bulletin, 1999) suggest that multifaceted interventions are required to effect change, although more research is required to focus on the effectiveness of specific interventions.

Our results (Thompson et al., 2000) suggest that there is potential in concentrating on the development of those sources of information that are used routinely in decision making, that is, human sources. The link nurse role (in operation at each of the study sites) would seem to be potentially valuable in the dissemination of information, although we need a better picture of how this operates nationally. To fulfil this function link nurses need to be supported by being given the resources they need (time, organisational and financial support) to carry out their role effectively.

Knowing about the types of decisions nurses make can assist nurse educators to integrate the teaching of decision making skills into all areas of the curriculum. As a fundamental first step, nurses need to be taught to recognise when a decision needs to be made (problem recognition and formulation). Results from the study based on the findings of one of the Q sorts suggest that nurses can be taught to rephrase a majority of their clinical decisions (concerning interventions and treatment) as clinical questions, for which they can then seek, appraise and apply research evidence in their practice (see Ch. 7 for further discussion of clinical questions). Nurses working together on a ward or unit could be encouraged to choose a decision that they face frequently (for example, 'should we shave patients prior to surgery or not?'), to turn it into a clinical question and to carry out the stages of evidence based practice in relation to this question. One way of storing the results of these efforts is as critically appraised topics (CATs; see http://cebm.jr2.ox.ac.uk/docs/cats/catabout.html). CATs are concise summaries of the evidence accompanied by a clinical 'bottom line' or take home message for clinicians. By using CATs in this way, a CAT bank of topics can be compiled (and updated regularly) to answer frequently occurring questions and assist with recurring decisions.

Nurse educators can also benefit from knowing how nurses interact with other professionals in negotiating joint decisions; they may wish to use role play as a tool to help nurses develop decision making skills that include negotiation with others.

Knowledge of the kinds of decisions nurses make is also fundamental to the development of decision aids (checklists, decision trees and other decision support initiatives). These types of decision aids are already in use in nursing, in areas such as 'walk in' facilities, or used to assist in triage in GP practices and accident and emergency departments (as well as NHS Direct). Finally, researchers need to further investigate nurse decision making as it actually occurs in different clinical contexts, using suitable methodologies. The decisions made by psychiatric nurses, community nurses and midwives will undoubtedly differ in some or many respects from those made by nurses in acute care, and are equally worthy of investigation.

CONCLUSION

A detailed knowledge of the types of decisions made routinely by nurses is a fundamental prerequisite for the development of an evidence base for nursing. The classification of actual decisions (as revealed through observation) into a decision typology provides a framework for the identification and structuring of 'real', that is, significant, clinical questions that require evidence from research.

Nurses should be given the opportunity to learn how to become effective decision makers from the very beginning of their training and throughout any professional education they undertake. Effective decision making should be highlighted in the curriculum as a crucial and integral component of the routine delivery of care by clinicians. To operate effectively as decision makers nurses need to acquire a range of skills, including:

◆ problem recognition
◆ forming clinical questions
◆ information retrieval
◆ risk assessment
◆ assessing resource implications
◆ negotiating with others (colleagues; patients; other professional groups)
◆ introducing and implementing change.

QUESTIONS FOR DISCUSSION

◆ How amenable is nurse decision making to research evidence?

◆ Which factors facilitate or hinder nurses in their use of research evidence?

◆ How may research findings be best disseminated to nurses so that they are incorporated routinely into daily practice?

◆ Are there areas of practice where nurses perceive a lack of research evidence? If so, where are they?

◆ How does decision making by community nurses differ from that of nurses working in the acute sector?

ANNOTATED FURTHER READING

Mulhall, A. & Le May, A. (eds) (1999). *Nursing research: Dissemination and implementation.* London: Churchill Livingstone.

This book addresses the question 'How can we ensure that the best research translates into best practice?'. It focuses on the theoretical and practical considerations behind the key issues of dissemination and implementation of research in nursing, and debates the critical issues raised.

Haines, A. & Donald, A. (eds) (1998). *Getting research findings into practice.* London: BMJ Publishing Group.

This accessible guide suggests ways of deciding whether findings should be implemented in practice and how to promote their uptake, and explains some of the possible reasons for failure. Topics covered include criteria for implementation, sources of information, behavioural factors and implementation, barriers to evidence, and decision analysis.

Bero, L., Grilli, R., Grimshaw, J., Harvey, E., Oxman, A., & Thompson, M.A. on behalf of the Cochrane Effective Practice and Organisation of Care Review Group (1998). Closing the gap between research and practice: an overview of systematic reviews of interventions to promote the implementation of research findings. *British Medical Journal, 317,* 465–468.

Many different types of intervention can be used to promote behavioural change among healthcare professionals and the implementation of research findings. This paper examines systematic reviews of different strategies for the dissemination and implementation of research findings to identify evidence of the effectiveness of different strategies and to assess the quality of the systematic reviews.

Bryans, A. & McIntosh, J. (1996). Decision making in community nursing: an analysis of the stages of decision making as they relate to community nursing assessment practice. *Journal of Advanced Nursing, 24,* 24–30.

This paper considers the nature of decisions made in the context of community nursing practice in the light of the stages of decision making distilled by Carroll & Johnson from the work of various theorists. It explores the relevance of each stage to community nurses' decision making.

REFERENCES

Benner, P. (1984). *From novice to expert: Excellence and power in clinical nursing practice.* Menlo Park, CA: Addison-Wesley.

Benner, P. & Tanner, C.A. (1987). Clinical judgement: How expert nurses use intuition. *American Journal of Nursing, 87*(1), 23–31.

Bucknall, T. (2000). Critical care nurses' decision-making activities in the natural clinical setting. *Journal of Clinical Nursing, 9,* 25–36.

Carr-Hill, R., Dixon, P., Gibbs, I. et al. (1992). *Skill mix and the effectiveness of nursing care.* York: Centre for Health Economics, University of York.

Cioffi, J. (2000). Nurses' experiences of making decisions to call emergency assistance to their patients. *Journal of Advanced Nursing, 32*(1), 108–114.

Crow, R., Chase, J., & Lamond, D. (1995). The cognitive component of nursing assessment: An analysis. *Journal of Advanced Nursing, 22,* 206–212.

Dunn, V., Crichton, N., Williams, K., Row, B., & Seers, K. (1998). Using research for practice: A UK experience of using the BARRIERS scale. *Journal of Advanced Nursing, 27,* 1203–1210.

Effective Health Care Bulletin (1999). *Getting evidence into practice.* York: NHS Centre for Reviews and Dissemination, University of York.

Funk, S.G., Tornquist, E.M., & Champagn, M.T. (1995). Barriers and facilitators of research utilization. *Nursing Clinics of North America, 30*(3), 395–407.

Jinks, A.M. & Hope, P. (2000). What do nurses do? An observational study of the activities of nurses on acute surgical and rehabilitation wards. *Journal of Nursing Management, 8*(5), 273–279.

Pyles, S.H. & Stern, P.N. (1983). Discovery of nursing gestalt in critical care nursing: The importance of the gray gorilla syndrome. *Image: The Journal of Nursing Scholarship, 15*(2), 51–57.

Schrader, B. & Fischer, D. (1987). Using intuitive knowledge in the neonatal intensive care nursery. *Holistic Nursing Practice, 1*(3), 45–51.

Thomas, L., McColl, E., Cullum, N., Rousseau, N., & Soutter, J. (1999). Clinical guidelines in nursing, midwifery and the therapies: A systematic review. *Journal of Advanced Nursing, 30*(1), 40–50.

Thompson, C., McCaughan, D., Cullum, N., Sheldon, T., & Thompson, D. (2000). *Nurses' use of research information in clinical decision making: A descriptive and analytical study – final report.* London: NCC SDO.

Watson, S. (1994). An exploratory study into a methodology for the examination of decision-making by nurses in the clinical area. *Journal of Advanced Nursing, 20,* 351–360.

Young, C. (1987). Intuition and the nursing process. *Holistic Nursing Practice, 1*(3), 52–56.

7

Making sense of research evidence to inform decision making

Kate Flemming   Mark Fenton

KEY ISSUES

◆ Making evidence based decisions means giving due weight to research evidence.

◆ Focused clinical questions can help reframe clinical uncertainty and in searching for evidence.

◆ Different sorts of research evidence 'fit' different sorts of clinical question and can be thought of hierarchically.

◆ Appraisal questions should be matched to the research design of the evidence.

◆ Numbers (measures of risk, harm, benefit and probability) can help establish what the clinical bottom line is for a piece of research.

CAVEAT

Evidence based health care has spawned a veritable library of texts and articles and a full and comprehensive treatment of the subject lies outside the scope of this book. This chapter is designed to act as an introduction to some of the major areas and to whet the reader's appetite for further study and exploration of the issues raised. To this end, we would strongly encourage readers to make use of the resources (both text based and online) detailed at the end of the chapter.

THE NATURE OF EVIDENCE

As Chapter 6 showed, the information sources nurses use to inform their decisions are varied. Nurses often make judgements and decisions based on several potentially flawed sources of information, such as the experience or expertise of oneself and others (Chs 2 and 6). These data sources for decision making are valuable but not when used alone or relied upon in isolation from broader (research) knowledge derived from hundreds, thousands or maybe millions of individuals receiving care and treatment. With the shift towards evidence based practice, nurses along with other health professionals, are being encouraged to put less emphasis on these 'flawed' sources of information and to place an appropriate weighting on research evidence when making decisions.

Sackett et al. (2000) define evidence based medicine (EBM) as '...the conscientious, explicit and judicious use of best evidence in making decisions about the care of individual patients. The practice of evidence based medicine means integrating individual clinical expertise with the best available external clinical evidence from systematic research'. This definition is applicable to all areas of health care – in fact, from now on we will refer to evidence based health care rather than evidence based medicine or evidence based nursing. Moreover, accepting this definition does not imply that medical approaches to care are somehow 'better' than a nursing approach (we are not sure that we could easily define what medical or nursing approaches to care really mean in practice anyway) or that different research designs are necessarily favoured or excluded. The evidence we need to make evidence based decisions is varied, as is the nature of the decisions we make in practice. This means we require different types of research evidence for different types of decisions.

The nature of research available for use in health care is ever changing and improving, as new research methodologies develop and new ways of understanding information become apparent. When asking questions of research, it is useful to know what types of evidence each type of research methodology can produce. There are two broad definitions of research methodology, quantitative and qualitative, each hiding a multitude of different approaches and providing different types of evidence to inform practice.

In general terms, quantitative research involves the collection of numeric types of information, whereas qualitative research collects more descriptive, naturalistic, types of information. These definitions do little to help the reader judge whether a research report is based on the most appropriate method for answering the questions posed or whether the study provides the appropriate evidence for the particular decision faced. To make these judgements, we must understand that the catch-all umbrella terms of quantitative and qualitative research contain a number of different designs. The next section explores these in more detail.

Quantitative research

The most often used quantitative methodologies in health care are case control studies, cohort studies and randomised controlled trials. Case control studies are used to try and ascertain the cause of a particular disease or condition. They firstly identify individuals with the disease or condition (cases) and then compare them to individuals who do not have the disease or condition. The starting point for cohort studies is exposure to a risk factor.

Descriptive cohort studies need a group of individuals who have been exposed to a risk factor (e.g. they live next to an electricity pylon). These individuals are then followed over a period of time to determine the incidence or frequency of the disease or condition of interest (e.g. childhood leukaemia). Sometimes the subjects of a descriptive cohort study are people who have the early stages of a disease and they are followed to observe the course of the disease over time (natural history studies).

In analytical cohort studies, we test the association between an exposure and an outcome. Study subjects are classified as exposed or unexposed to the risk factor of interest and then followed over a period of time to see whether they develop one or more outcomes (e.g. you have a cohort of smokers and non-smokers and follow them up over a period of years to see if they develop lung cancer).

Randomised controlled trials (RCTs) are used to try to assess the effectiveness of a treatment or intervention (e.g. whether a new wound dressing is more effective in healing chronic leg ulcers than conventional care). In an RCT the researcher randomly allocates one group of subjects to the 'treatment' group, and these subjects receive the treatment under investigation (the new wound dressing). A second group of subjects is allocated to the 'control' group and do not receive the intervention (such as an existing dressing regimen). Both groups are then followed over a period of time to see whether they develop the outcome(s) of interest (e.g. their leg ulcers heal faster with the new wound dressing). A control group is required so that the outcomes in the intervention group can be compared with those in the control group (Gordis, 1996). The crucial advantage of a randomised controlled trial is that where a difference occurs between control and intervention groups, and where the study is large enough and of good enough quality, then we can be more confident than with non-randomised approaches that the observed difference is really due to the intervention as opposed to chance.

Qualitative research

Qualitative studies are used to try and understand or describe the feelings and perceptions of individuals. In health care these studies often examine how individuals live or cope with a particular disease or with a particular treatment (e.g. how does it feel to live with four layer bandaging techniques, as a treatment for leg ulcers?). Qualitative studies draw on a wide variety of philosophical and academic schools (anthropology, ethnography, phenomenology). However, the most common kinds of data in qualitative studies are observed behaviours and interview material. The data is then examined systematically and rigorously to identify common themes amongst those observed and/or interviewed. In qualitative research it is not always necessary to have comparisons between groups because it is the description or explanation of phenomena that is often the focus, rather than the extrapolation of generalisable differences between experimental and control groups.

This section has been (necessarily) brief and readers are directed to the more detailed texts on qualitative research, some of which explore its role in evidence based health care, indicated at the end of the chapter.

A note on the quality of evidence and thinking hierarchically

A common misconception among nurses is that the only kind of research that counts in evidence based decision making is RCTs – this is wrong. If the uncertainty that you face in a decision centres on which one of two or more options is likely to prove most beneficial to the patient then RCTs do indeed provide the most valuable form of research evidence. Even better than the results of one RCT are the results of lots of similar RCTs, all reviewed systematically, to come up with a definitive and more accurate picture.

So RCTs are great when you need to know 'what works best' but no RCT will ever act as the best source of information if you need to know 'how people might feel about a particular intervention' (qualitative or survey approaches are the most useful) or 'what happens to people newly diagnosed with diabetes who are left untreated?' (cohort studies are the best approach here).

The (oft referred to) hierarchy of evidence (Fig. 7.1) is an attempt to represent a very simple idea: that for particular kinds of knowledge needs in decisions there are particular, complementary, research designs. As you move down the hierarchy the chances of reaching reliable, accurate and unbiased answers decrease. Systematic reviews of RCTs (for questions of effectiveness – or what works best) are at the top of the hierarchy because they rigorously summarise all the studies that have been done on a topic. RCTs are next because, when properly conducted, they minimise biases such as selection bias (where the treatment a patient receives is not necessarily determined by chance but may be determined by how well the researcher believes the patient will do on that treatment).

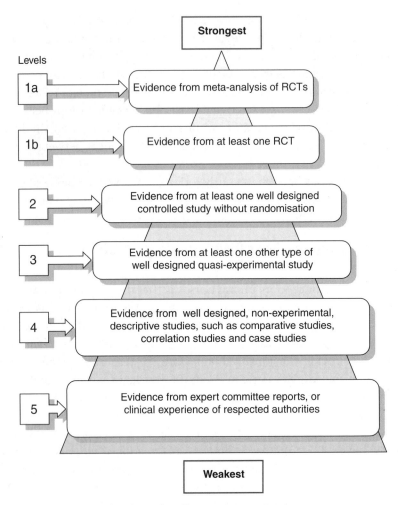

Figure 7.1 Hierarchy of evidence for effectiveness questions.

EVIDENCE BASED DECISIONS

There are four main influences in an evidence based decision (Fig. 7.2):

◆ clinical experience
◆ research evidence
◆ patient preference
◆ available resources.

Critics of evidence based health care often make claims that the approach fosters a 'cook book' approach to decision making, urging practitioners to neglect the circumstances surrounding a decision or negating

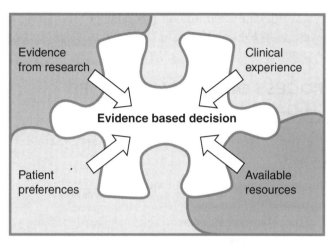

Figure 7.2 The four components of an evidence based decision.

the practitioner's existing knowledge. By acknowledging that there are four parts to any evidence based decision, some of these criticisms are countered. In different circumstances, different weight can be given to each part of the jigsaw. For example, take a situation where the research evidence advises parents of babies under the age of 1 year to put them to sleep on their backs. However, the clinical experience of a health visitor may outweigh this research evidence when advising a parent of a baby with a cardiac condition that in this instance implementing the research evidence is inappropriate given the other circumstances (the cardiac condition) that need to be considered. Similarly, in the case of a patient with multiple sclerosis, the patient might request treatment with beta interferon, the clinical experience of the nurse may favour its use and the research evidence found by the nurse may support its use but the resources are not there to prescribe the course of treatment. In this situation the available resources outweigh all other aspects of the decision jigsaw.

 Examining definitions of evidence based health care reinforces the idea that there are multiple elements to the decision making process, for example Hicks (1997) states: 'evidence based health care takes place when decisions that affect the care of patients are taken with due weight accorded to all valid relevant information'. Whilst Gray (1997) defines evidence based clinical practice as ' ... an approach to decision making in which the clinician uses the best evidence available, in consultation with the patient, to decide the option that suits the patient best'.

In today's health care environment it is only by considering all the elements relevant to a decision that an evidence based decision can be said to have been made.

THE PROCESS OF EVIDENCE BASED HEALTH CARE

To practise evidence based health care, practitioners need to develop skills in six key stages:

◆ reviewing practice and identifying uncertainty
◆ phrasing answerable questions
◆ searching for research evidence
◆ critical appraisal of the research – what should we be doing?
◆ implementation (where appropriate)
◆ audit – what are we doing?

Each of these processes will be examined in turn.

Stage one – reviewing practice and identifying uncertainty

In busy, everyday practice it is easy to continue what one has been doing in an unquestioning manner with the 'certainty' that the decisions you take will deliver optimal benefits to the patient. However, it is important to maintain an open mind and to distinguish between what one believes to be true and what is actually true. A number of opportunities exist for fostering this open mindedness. One of the best opportunities to reflect on everyday practice is when an 'outsider', for example, a student or visitor, observes practice and questions what might otherwise be seen as routine. Practitioners can also encounter new situations that immediately alert them to gaps in their knowledge – these might include being confronted with an unusual condition, disease or situation, or could arise because a patient has discovered new information about the condition he or she is suffering and is seeking to establish its veracity.

Whatever the situation about which information is sought, it is vital that the uncertainty that brought it about in the first place is managed. This is the next stage in the evidence based process of decision making.

Stage two – phrasing answerable questions

The reflection that arises from stage one must be clearly formulated into a question to ensure clear answers are obtained from literature searching.

Producing focused questions maximises scarce searching time whilst ensuring that the practitioner has considered (and narrowed down) the information being sought.

A way of developing a focused question is by formulating it in such a way that it reflects the topic of interest. The focused question then becomes the centre of the search strategy. Questions generally have three elements to them:

◆ the situation, population or person
◆ the intervention
◆ the outcome.

The situation, population or person you are interested in

Evidence based health care involves defining the patient as a member of a population in terms of clinical problem, age, sex, ethnic group, and so on. However, it could also deal with any aspect of health care delivery, for example, 'how is the distribution of pressure relieving devices organised within an acute trust?' 'how are appointments managed?'.

High quality research papers should be explicit in describing the criteria used to select subjects. Often, however, the participants in a study do not exactly match those identified by the searcher so one of the key questions to ask of papers retrieved from a search is 'Are the subjects in this study so different from my situation that I cannot generalise its findings?'.

The intervention

This is the plan being considered or the current intervention that requires assessing. Interventions can be a number of things for example: a type of therapy (e.g. choice of wound dressing, selection of pharmaceutical product), some preventative measure (e.g. counselling on lifestyle and risk factors), a diagnostic measure (e.g. which patients should have blood pressure measured and how often?) or a management issue (e.g. when to refer patients on to other professionals).

A comparator is often required to determine whether or not one of two (or more) possible interventions is better than the other. This is particularly the case with questions of therapy: it might be that current treatment for leg ulcers is Una's boot but a comparison with four layer compression bandaging is required because this is being suggested as a new form of treatment.

The outcome(s)

Outcomes are the end point of interest arising from the intervention being investigated. From the example above, when Una's boot was being compared with four layered bandaging the outcome of interest might have been ulcer healing or reduction in ulcer size. The outcome is entirely dependent on the question, which in turn stems from professional practice.

Ideally, research papers should specify the end point they are measuring, which will help in selecting relevant ones. However it is sometimes necessary to read between the lines of a paper to work out what the authors are actually trying to prove.

Stage three – searching for research evidence

The type of papers that are looked for and the places searched depend on the nature of the question being asked. A broad range of possible questions can arise from nursing practice:

◆ communication (how do we best communicate information to patients?)
◆ feelings, perceptions (how is somebody likely to feel in this situation?)
◆ therapies (which works best – intervention X or intervention Y?)
◆ prevention (how can I stop my patients developing sacral pressure sores?)
◆ prognosis (what are the chances of developing diabetes after myocardial infarct?)
◆ causation/harm (do deep vein thromboses lead to leg ulcers?)
◆ organisation of services (what's the best way of setting up a coordinated discharge scheme?)

When searching, the best available evidence for a particular question needs identifying. Table 7.1 identifies types of research or evidence that match types of clinical or managerial questions.

Sources of evidence available

A huge number of sources of evidence is available to search, including textbooks, journals, bibliographic databases, distilled and condensed information sources, and the Internet.

Textbooks are most useful for accessing 'stable information' such as anatomy and physiology and the pathology of illness. It is worth bearing in mind when consulting a textbook that information is often at least 2 years old at the point of publishing and that it might contain many unreferenced sources.

Table 7.1 How evidence relates to questions about practice

Type of question	Example	Best evidence from
Effectiveness of treatment/ prevention; adverse effects of treatments	Does compression bandaging increase the healing of venous leg ulcers compared with no compression?	Results of systematic literature reviews or meta-analyses based on randomised controlled trials
Causation	Are people who have had a deep vein thrombosis more likely to get a leg ulcer than people who have not?	Results of systematic literature reviews or meta-analyses based on cohort studies
Feelings; understandings; perceptions	How do people with venous leg ulcers feel about their health and their lifestyle?	Qualitative studies

There is a huge number of journals available. However, different journals meet different needs. Points to bear in mind when considering a journal include whether it is peer reviewed, what scope it has (local, national or international) and whether it reports research findings or more general news. Generally, nursing journals report on advances in research and practice, whilst major health care advances are reported in general medical journals. Journals do have the disadvantage of potential publication bias and differ in the length of time between receiving a paper and publishing it. In general, reading individual journals is not an efficient way of answering specific questions.

Many bibliographic databases are now available for searching. Two of the most commonly used for accessing nursing information are the Cumulated Index to Nursing and Allied Health Literature (CINAHL), which contains over quarter of a million articles from over 650 English language journals, and MEDLINE, which contains articles indexed from more than 3500 journals.

A number of distilled information resources are also particularly relevant to evidence based health care. These resources are journals that review other journals and select only relevant, high quality research studies from these and produce a critical appraisal and clinical commentary of the work presented. Examples of such journals are *Evidence Based Nursing*, *Evidence Based Medicine* and *Evidence Based Mental Health*. You can access the contents pages and full text of (some of) these journals via the worldwide web.

Consolidated information sources contain systematic reviews of the results of a number of research studies. The primary resource for finding systematic reviews is the Cochrane library (http://www.cochranelibrary.com). The Cochrane Library is actually four databases:

◆ Cochrane Database of Systematic Reviews: a database of systematic reviews and planned reviews carried out for the Cochrane Collaboration.
◆ Database of Abstracts of Reviews of Effectiveness (DARE): critically appraised abstracts of systematic reviews. The abstracts are produced by reviewers from the NHS Centre for Reviews and Dissemination at the University of York.
◆ Cochrane Review Methodology Update: articles, links and resources for those considering or undertaking a review.
◆ Cochrane Controlled Trials Register: a register of controlled trials identified by reviewers for the Cochrane Collaboration.

Hundreds of valuable information sources are available on the Internet. However, they are not appraised for quality and therefore need to be used with caution. Increasingly, bibliographic databases and journal contents can be accessed free via the worldwide web. The Internet is a resource available for everyone and is more frequently being accessed by patients to gain information regarding their healthcare status. Useful web addresses for accessing information are given in the Annotated further reading section at the end of the chapter.

Stage four – appraisal of information retrieved

There is a huge variation in quality in the research evidence that is available. For this reason it is essential to critically appraise any research obtained; using inaccurate or unreliable evidence is probably worse than not using evidence at all. We need to determine whether we can trust the results of a research paper in order to decide if it is appropriate to apply the findings to our practice. It is beyond the scope of this chapter to examine the appraisal techniques of each of the research methods that are commonly used in nursing and healthcare research because each research design merits a different set of appraisal questions. Some online and literary resources that will point you in the direction of appropriate appraisal checklists are presented in the Annotated further reading section. However, some basic questions can be asked of any paper in order to determine the accuracy of the claimed results. The series of questions in Box 7.1 should be asked of all research papers, irrespective of which

> **Box 7.1** Appraisal questions to ask of all research papers
>
> ◆ Is the focus of the research clearly stated?
> ◆ Can the research population be generalised to your own client group?
> ◆ Was the sample size justified?
> ◆ Are any measurement tools used valid and reliable?
> ◆ Did untoward events occur during the study?
> ◆ Were the basic data adequately described?
> ◆ Do the numbers add up?
> ◆ What do the main findings mean?
> ◆ How do the results compare with previous reports?
> ◆ Have the authors overlooked any issues that you consider to be important?
> ◆ What implications does the study have for your practice?
>
> (Crombie, 1996)

method has been used. They are a good starting point for appraising the quality of research papers.

Interpreting the results of research

Results from research (using either quantitative or qualitative methods) can be difficult to interpret and translate into something clinically meaningful. However, some simple rules allow the reader to make some sense of reported results. First, we will consider the interpretation of results from single quantitative research studies, followed by ways of interpreting the results from systematic reviews and meta-analyses.

There are several types of results used to report outcomes in research, these range from proportions of participants who experience an event (better to not better, experienced side effects to did not experience side effects), to the difference between two average (mean) scores taken from a rating scale, plus many other ways of reporting statistical outcomes. In research that reports results of an experiment, the type of summary statistic we need to see is one of impact: how different is one intervention over another in changing a specific outcome (such as better or not better). In qualitative research that is exploring a question such as 'what is it like to live with a chronic disease?' we would want to see a topic or a theme reported consistently by many of the participants independently of each other.

Results from single studies The aim of providing results of statistical testing in a research report is to estimate the probability that the results found in a sample of participants are valid, that is, they did not occur simply by chance. Just as importantly, the clinician has to interpret whether statistical significance equates to a clinically significant result. The results of statistical testing are often given in the form of p-values. p-values, (sometimes seen as $p > 0.05$ or $p < 0.05$), are a measure of probability and allow the reader to decide whether a result has arisen as a result of the treatment or intervention, or by chance.

Probability can be explained by thinking of a die. If you throw a die, there is a one in six chance that the next number to come up will be a six. This can be expressed as 1/6 or 0.166 or 16.6%. When a p-value is given in reports of research, it generally refers to the probability that the results did not occur by chance. The conventional cut-off point for deciding that the results are not due to chance is a one in twenty probability that the results occurred by chance (think of a twenty-sided die). This means that a result has to have less than or equal to a 0.05 chance of occurring by chance alone (expressed as $p = 0.05$). This 0.05 cut off is arbitrary but is the accepted level for considering whether a result is statistically significant or not. p-values of 0.05 or less are said to be significant, 0.01 or less highly significant and above 0.05 (e.g. 0.06 and closer to 1), as not statistically significant (this does not mean, however, that they are of no clinical importance). For instance, say you carried out a randomised controlled trial comparing Una's boot with four layer compression bandaging for the treatment of leg ulcers. After carrying out statistical testing, it appears that the bandaging system is 'better' at healing ulcers, with a statistical significance of $p < 0.05$. This means that it is highly likely (or probable) that the results of your experiment were because of the intervention (there is only a 5% probability that this result happened by chance).

It also needs to be remembered that statistical significance is different to clinical significance:

Researchers and readers of research often focus excessively on whether a result is statistically significant (i.e. not likely the result of chance). However, just because a test shows a treatment effect to be statistically significant, it does not mean the result is clinically important. For example, if a study is very large (and therefore has a small standard error), it is easier to find small and clinically unimportant treatment effects to be statistically significant. A large randomised controlled trial compared rehospitalisations in patients receiving a new heart drug with patients *receiving usual care. A 1% reduction in rehospitalisations was reported in the treatment group (49% rehospitalisations v 50% in the usual care group). This was highly statistically significant (p < 0.0001) mainly because this is a large trial. However, it is unlikely that clinical practice would be changed on the basis of such a small reduction in hospitalisation.* (Sheldon, 2000)

Results from systematic reviews and meta-analyses This section deals with interpreting and translating results reported in systematic reviews or meta-analyses. The following ways of reporting are all based on comparisons between two groups and the result being reported discretely (i.e. the patient improved or not; died or did not die). It is beyond the scope of this chapter to explore fully the interpretation of continuous data (i.e. that measured on a continuous scale, such as blood pressure). By comparing the results of two groups, the aim is to estimate whether there is a difference in the outcomes found in either. It is the difference between these two results that allows clinicians and others to say a new intervention is, or is not, an improvement on the standard treatment, or groups with certain characteristics are more prone to a certain disease than groups without those characteristics.

However, the way results are reported can be confusing. What is the clinical meaning of a 10% change on a rating scale, or a mean difference of 0.03 between two (or more) groups? It is important to note that different types of research calculate the same outcome in different ways. There are a number of ways in which the differences in results between two groups are reported. These include (Henry et al., 1997):

◆ *Relative risk* – the risk for achieving an outcome in the treatment group relative to that in the control group.
◆ *Relative risk reduction (RRR)* – the increase in outcome with the treatment compared to the control (often expressed as a percentage).
◆ *Absolute risk reduction (ARR)* – the difference in outcome rates for two groups, usually treatment and control.
◆ *Number needed to treat (NNT)* – the number of persons who must be treated for a given period to achieve an outcome.
◆ *Odds ratio* – the number of events relative to the number of non-events (the odds of an event in the treatment group divided by the odds of an event in the comparison group).

An example will help illustrate the differences in the different types of reporting of results. The results of a prospective study on the incidence

Table 7.2 Summary of results from Vyhlidal et al. (1997)

Outcome	Mattress EER (%)	Overlay CER (%)	RRR (%) (95% CI)	ARR (%)	NNT (%) (95% CI)
Patients with pressure sores	25	60	58 (10 to 82)	35	3 (2 to 23)

ARR, absolute risk reduction; CER, control event rate; CI, confidence interval; EER, experimental event rate; NNT, number needed to treat; RRR, relative risk reduction.

of pressure sores associated with nursing patients on a foam mattress replacement versus a foam overlay (Vyhlidal et al., 1997) are reported in Table 7.2. These results indicate that in the individuals who had a foam mattress, 25% (0.25) of patients developed pressure sores compared to 60% (0.6) of patients who had a foam overlay. These results can be reported in a number of different ways, some of which are presented already in the table.

In this instance, the relative risk of developing pressure sores is the risk in the treatment (mattress) group relative to that of the control (foam group). This is calculated by dividing the risk in the treatment group by that of the control ($0.25 \div 0.6 = 0.42$). This indicates that if you are treated with a foam mattress you are 42% (0.42) less likely to develop pressure sores than if you were treated with a foam overlay. The relative risk reduction is the ratio between the decrease in risk in the mattress group and the risk in the foam group (the decrease in risk is $0.6 - 0.25 = 0.35$, so the relative risk reduction is $0.35 \div 0.6 = 0.58$ or 58% – as indicated in Table 7.2). This means there was a relative reduction of 58% (0.58) in pressure sores in the group treated with foam mattress. The problem with both relative risk and relative risk reduction is that the value is the same regardless of the clinical significance of changes in risk (e.g. a reduction of $0.6 - 0.25$ has the same relative risk as that of $0.00063 - 0.0015$) (Henry et al., 1997). For this reason, results are often given in the form of an absolute risk reduction, which is determined by subtracting the absolute risk in the treatment group (mattress) from the risk in the control group ($0.6 - 0.25 = 0.35$, or 35%). This means that among those individuals who had a foam mattress there were 35% fewer instances of pressure sore development than those who were treated with foam overlay.

Results are often presented in terms of the number needed to treat. The NNT indicates the number of people you need to treat with a particular intervention to achieve your desired outcome, over a specific period of time. The NNT is the reciprocal of the ARR (the NNT for the above example is $1 \div 0.35 = 2.85$, or 3 – as in Table 7.2). This indicates that you need to treat three people with a foam mattress to prevent one person from developing pressure sores. With the NNT, a small value means that a favourable outcome occurs in nearly every person who has the treatment. It is inappropriate to compare NNTs across disease conditions (Henry et al., 1997) because it is a treatment-specific value. However, you can compare NNTs for different interventions for the same condition and same outcome. This allows you to compare the relative effectiveness of different treatment interventions for the same condition (Henry et al., 1997).

Finally, you may often see the results of research presented as odds ratios (OR). The odds ratio is a reference to the odds of the event happening in one group compared to another group (Gordis, 1996). Examples of events are things like better versus not better, side effect versus no side effect, has a disease versus does not have disease.

A summary of Maisel and Kring (1998) in *Evidence Based Nursing* reported a study that examined 127 infants readmitted to hospital within 14 days of discharge compared against 127 babies who were also discharged during the same period but not readmitted. The study aimed to identify risk factors for those children most at risk of readmission to hospital following discharge and compare the frequency that the risk factor occurred in the readmitted group against the frequency in the group that was not readmitted. The summary reports the odds ratio of being readmitted as being highest for those children whose gestational age was less than or equal to 36 weeks, having jaundice in the nursery prior to discharge, being between 36 and 37 weeks gestational age, and being breastfed. Table 7.3 is reproduced from the summary. In those children whose gestational age was ≤36 weeks, the odds of being readmitted were 13.2 times greater than for those whose gestational age was >36 weeks. When we look at gestational age being >40 weeks, we can see the OR is 0.4. This could be considered to be a demonstration of a protective effect of gestational age upon the odds of being readmitted (because an odds ratio of 1 represents no difference in risk between the two groups; Box 7.2).

You might also have noticed that some of the results in Tables 7.2 and 7.3 also present a confidence interval (CI). This quantifies the uncertainty in the measurement. A 95% CI reports the range of values within which we can be 95% sure that the true (population) value lies. For instance, in Table 7.2 the 95% CI for the relative risk reduction (RRR) is 10–82%.

Table 7.3 Risk factors for infant hospital readmission for hyperbilirubinaemia – summary of results from Maisel and Kring (1998)

Variables	Study group (%)	Control group (%)	Odds ratio (95% CI)
Gestational age ≤ 36 weeks	9.5	1.6	13.2 (2.7 to 64.6)
Jaundice in nursery	90.6	55.9	7.8 (3.4 to 18.0)
Gestational age 36–37 weeks	16.5	4.7	7.7 (2.7 to 22.0)
Gestational age 37–38 weeks	28.4	8.7	7.2 (3.1 to 17.0)
Breast feeding	89.0	63.8	4.2 (1.8 to 9.9)
Length of stay	47.1	33.1	3.2 (1.4 to 7.1)
Male sex	74.8	49.6	2.9 (1.5 to 5.7)
Length of stay <48 hours	47.2	46.5	2.4 (1.1 to 5.3)
Gestational age >40 weeks	15.8	34.7	0.4 (0.2 to 0.7)
Initial length of stay >72 hours	8.7	20.5	0.4 (0.2 to 0.8)
No meconium	3.2	22.8	0.2 (0.04 to 0.6)
Rupture of membranes >18 hours before birth	1.6	7.1	0.08 (0.01 to 0.5)

Box 7.2 A general interpretation of the odds ratio

◆ OR = 1: there is no difference between the groups, therefore no risk.

◆ OR > 1: there is a greater risk for those who have this outcome (variable).

◆ OR < 1: the risk is decreased for those with this outcome, suggesting a possible protective effect.

This means we are 95% certain that the mattress reduces the incidence of pressure sores by 10–82%. Similarly, in Table 7.3 the CI for the odds ratio for gestational age ≤ 36 weeks was 2.7–64.6. This means that if the baby was less than 36 weeks old we are 95% certain he or she will have increased odds of being readmitted of between 2.7 times greater to 64.6 times greater, than a child over 36 weeks gestation. The large range of these figures is worth noting here. Clearly, with regard to the incidence of pressure sores, there is a significant clinical difference between a reduction of 10% and one of 82%. In this case, the nurse would have to weigh up the financial and nursing implications involved in adopting decision choices when the risk reduction might only be in the order of 1 in 10 against the more optimistic picture of 1 in 1.12.

Stage five – implementation

The implementation of evidence based practice is one of the most difficult and complex areas of the whole process. It is relatively easy for the individual practitioner to change his or her own practice, however, practitioners rarely operate in such isolation that a change in their own practice will not have an influence on that of their colleagues. As such, implementing evidence based practice is synonymous with the processes of change management.

A systematic review of the research evidence for interventions aimed at getting evidence into practice (NHS Centre for Reviews and Dissemination, 1999) made the following recommendations:

◆ A range of interventions has been shown to be effective in changing professional behaviour in some circumstances. Multifaceted interventions targeting different barriers to change are more likely to be effective than single interventions.
◆ Successful strategies to change practice need to be resourced adequately and require people with appropriate knowledge and skills.
◆ Any systematic approach to changing professional practice should include plans to monitor and evaluate and to maintain and reinforce any change.

The basic messages for implementing change are that no one single method is most effective in producing change and that a considered number of approaches relevant to the local area should be employed. In addition to this, appropriate personnel with local knowledge and the time and resources to fully carry out the task are required, otherwise the process of change is likely to fail.

Stage six – audit

Evaluation of the process of implementing evidence based practice is vital to determine whether changes have influenced practice and, ultimately, patient care. Limited space and scope preclude a detailed discussion of clinical audit and its role in evidence based health care here. However, there are a number of clear and useful texts on the subject and the reader is strongly encouraged to make use of the links in the Annotated further reading section at the end of the chapter.

It is worth remembering that the process of clinical audit is cyclical. Whilst definitions of audit are multifarious and not terribly helpful (Crombie et al., 1997), one characteristic that all approaches share is that practitioner effort during clinical audit should focus on fulfilling the key stages of an audit cycle. The basic audit stages of observing current practice, setting standards of care, comparing practice with the standards and implementing a change should be addressed in a continuous and iterative way. There should be no predetermined end point for stopping the cycle.

CONCLUSION

This chapter has examined how research evidence can be incorporated within clinical decision making. To ensure that your decision making is based on the 'best' evidence, you need to know how to search for evidence and to be able to interpret what the results of studies mean. However, research evidence is only one of a number of different types of 'evidence' you can use to make decisions. You need to be clear when (and if) the research you use is appropriate for your decision making. However, only a brief excursion into a much bigger literature has been possible here. If the chapter has whet your appetite, we would encourage you to explore further.

QUESTIONS FOR DISCUSSION

◆ How much of your practice is *really* evidence based?

◆ What are the common questions that arise from your practice and can you convert these into focused clinical questions?

◆ Can you establish which are the most pressing questions requiring evidence based answers?

◆ What facilities exist for you to be able to make progress towards evidence based health care decision making?

◆ How might you make best use of these facilities: (i) as an individual and (ii) as a team or unit?

◆ Do you *really* know how to appraise a research paper so that you can give its results due weight in your decision making?

ANNOTATED FURTHER READING

The 'must visit' site has to be SCHARR's excellent web resources page at http://www.shef.ac.uk/~scharr/links.htm especially good is the 'netting the evidence' section, which provides links to appraisal sheets, search filters and online training.

If you just want to get searching quickly then the University of Rochester's evidence based search filters are useful (and easily adapted to whatever front end software you use, such as Silverplatter or PUBMED): http://www.urmc.rochester.edu/Miner/Educ/Expertsearch.html

If you are not new to evidence based health care and feel ready to start calculating some numbers to help you give due weight to research evidence, or if you want to revise some probabilities, then the excellent family medicine site is for you; it has more calculators and spreadsheets than you are ever likely to need: http://www.fammed.ouhsc.edu/robhamm/cdmcalc.htm

For the traditionalists, good starting points for paper based reading include:

Sackett, D., Strauss, S.E., Richardson, W.S., Rosenburg, W., & Haynes, R.B. (2000). *Evidence based medicine: How to practice and teach EBM*. London: Churchill Livingstone.

For a more detailed treatment of clinical audit have a look at:

Crombie, I.K., Davies, H.T.O., Abraham S.C.S., & Flare C.Du.V. (1997). *The audit handbook: Improving health care through clinical audit*. London: John Wiley.

An all round introduction to appraisal aimed at nurses was written by the team at the Centre for Evidence Based Nursing and published in *Nursing Time's* Learning Curve Series between March and November, 1999. (*Nursing Times 3* (1–9)).

REFERENCES

Crombie, I.K. (1996). *The pocket guide to critical appraisal*. London: BMJ Publishing.
Crombie, I.K., Davies, H.T.O., Abraham S.C.S., & Flare, C.Du.V. (1997). *The audit handbook: Improving health care through clinical audit*. London: John Wiley.
Gordis, L. (1996). *Epidemiology*. Philadelphia: W.B. Saunders.
Gray, J.A.M. (1997). *Evidence based health care: How to make health policy and management decisions*. Edinburgh: Churchill Livingstone.
Henry, J., McQuay, D.M., & Moore, R.A. (1997). Using numerical results from systematic reviews in clinical practice. *Annals of Internal Medicine, 126*(1 May), 712–720.
Hicks, N. (1997). Evidence based health care. *Bandolier, 4*(39), 8.
Maisel, M.J. & Kring, E. (1998). Length of stay, jaundice and hospital readmission. *Pediatrics* (June), 995–998.
NHS Centre for Reviews and Dissemination (1999). *Effective health care: Getting evidence into practice*. London: Royal Society of Medicine Press Ltd.
Sackett, D.L., Richardson, S.W., Rosenberg, W., & Haynes, R.B. (2000). *Evidence-based medicine: How to practice and teach EBM*. London: Churchill Livingstone.
Sheldon, T.A. (2000). Estimating treatment effects: Real or the result of chance? *Evidence-Based Nursing, 3*, 36–39.
Vyhlidal, S.K., Moxness, D., Bosak, K.S. et al. (1997). Mattress replacement or foam overlay? A prospective study on the incidence of pressure sores. *Applied Nursing Research, 10*, 111–120.

8

Decision analysis

Dawn Dowding   Carl Thompson

KEY ISSUES

◆ Decision analysis is a rational and prescriptive model of decision
  support.

◆ Decision analysis helps maximise the utility of individuals
  receiving health care.

◆ Decision analysis is especially useful for treatment- or
  effectiveness-type decisions.

Up to this point in the book we have discussed decision making in a rather abstract way. This is the first in a series of more 'applied' chapters that discuss ways in which decision making can be improved in practice. This chapter provides an overview of decision analysis – one technique for applying a more rational approach to decisions. In doing so, we highlight the particular benefits and limitations of the approach.

WHAT IS DECISION ANALYSIS?

Decision analysis is a prescriptive model of decision making, meaning that it is trying to 'improve' how individuals make decisions (Chapman & Sonnenberg, 2000). It relies on the premise that humans should choose models of decision making that are logical and rational. In the language of decision making theory and economics, the approach tries to maximise individuals' 'expected utility' by helping steer them towards the best decision choice (i.e. one that fits their beliefs or values most appropriately). Decision analysis is used only in conditions of uncertainty, a concept that you should by now be familiar with. It is also only really useful for complex decisions, where the optimum decision option is not always obvious.

Decision analysis works by breaking a decision down into a number of choices, adding numerical values (usually the probability of events) to each part of the decision situation, and then calculating which option has the highest utility for the decision maker.

> *Clinical decision analysis uses… techniques to make the decision making process explicit, it also breaks down the process into its component parts so that the effect of using different observations, actions, probabilities and utilities can be analysed.*
> (Llewelyn & Hopkins, 1993)

Clinical problems or decisions are usually constructed as a decision tree (Dowie, 1996). These schematic representations usually follow a natural timeline from left to right (i.e. the first event and decision choice at the left through to the last on the right). Decision analysts are required to clearly separate the choices or options open to the individual, the chances or uncertainties that may occur as a result of the different options and the different outcomes that may arise (Dowie, 1996). Figure 8.1 shows a typical decision tree. The different decision options are shown as square nodes, the chance events that can occur as a result of these decisions as circle nodes and triangle nodes represent the outcomes of chance events. Attached to the decision tree is the probability, or likelihood, of a chance

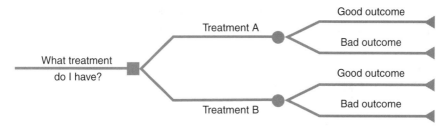

Figure 8.1 Basic structure of a decision tree.

event occurring, together with the value or utility the person attaches to each outcome, as a numerical value.

CARRYING OUT A DECISION ANALYSIS

The best way of illustrating how decision analysis works is by considering a clinical decision problem. The example in Scenario 8.1 is based on work by Pauker and Pauker (1977) and is discussed by Dowie (1992).

Scenario 8.1

You are a midwife in an antenatal clinic and have before you a 40-year-old woman, pregnant with her first child. She is at 'high' risk of having a baby with some form of genetic abnormality, such as Downs syndrome. She needs to decide whether to have a test to see whether her baby has a potential problem. She has the choice of two different tests, a chorion villus sampling (CVS) test or an amniocentesis. The CVS can be carried out earlier in her pregnancy than the amniocentesis and, if the tests come back positive, then it is assumed that she will have an abortion. This means that if she has a CVS she is likely to terminate the pregnancy at an earlier stage than if she has an amniocentesis (with the potential psychological benefits this carries). However, both tests carry a risk of spontaneous abortion or miscarriage and they are not 100% accurate. How could you help this woman make a decision regarding what to do?

Decision analysis has been used in practice to try and help women make such decisions (Pauker & Pauker, 1977). It is a decision made under uncertainty, as there are a variety of different outcomes that may happen if the woman agrees or does not agree to a test (such as positive and negative results or miscarriage). The values the woman attaches to the different outcomes also need to be taken into account.

Step one – structuring the tree

Doubilet and McNeil (1988) suggest that when structuring a decision problem there is a need for compromise between simplifying the problem too much and including enough detail for it to be relevant. Tree structures are often designed in consultation with an expert in the clinical field, so that all relevant options are considered without the tree becoming too detailed. As an example, a possible structure for the decision problem in Scenario 8.1 is shown in Figure 8.2. This indicates that the woman has three choices: to not have a test at all, to have a CVS or to have an amniocentesis test (represented by the square node). Depending on which option she chooses, different chance events or outcomes can occur. For example, if she chooses not to have a test, there is a chance (probability) that she may have a miscarriage anyway. Or, there is a probability that her pregnancy will continue to term, after which she might (or might not) have a child affected with a genetic abnormality. If she chooses to have a test she may spontaneously abort as a result, or the test results will come back either positive or negative. If the result is positive, then (for the purpose of this model) she would have an elective abortion. If it is negative, her pregnancy will (again for the purposes of the example) proceed to term. Added into this model is the possibility that despite a negative result the baby may have a genetic abnormality (false negative), something that

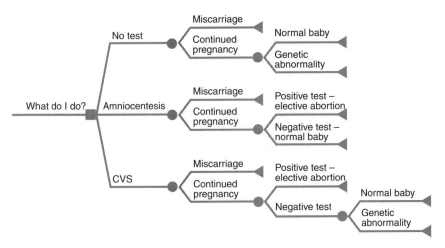

Figure 8.2 Structure for the prenatal testing decision.

you should be aware of after the discussions regarding test results in Chapters 2 and 5.

Step two – assessing probability

The second stage in the analysis is to work out the probability or likelihood of the events happening for each decision choice – or branch – of the tree. Probabilities can be obtained from 'objective' data, such as epidemiological or research studies. Indeed, this is one of the ways in which results from research findings can be applied to clinical decisions. However, when there is no research evidence for the different chance options, subjective data can be used instead, such as expert estimations of the likelihood of an event happening (Panniers & Walker, 1994). The point of the decision tree is to foster a logical approach to option selection – it does not rely on research evidence for its success.

For the purposes of the example, assume that the probabilities of the outcomes occurring are as follows (these figures have been derived from information provided to women by the Glasgow Royal Maternity Hospital and a systematic review carried out by Alfirevic et al. (2000)):

◆ the prevalence of chromosome abnormality in the babies of this group of women is 1.7%
◆ amniocentesis has a sensitivity of 99.9% and specificity of 100%
◆ CVS has a sensitivity of 99.4% and a specificity of 99.8%
◆ the probability of a 40-year-old woman in her first pregnancy having a spontaneous abortion/miscarriage is 0.5%
◆ the probability of having a miscarriage after an amniocentesis test is 1%
◆ the probability of having a miscarriage after a CVS is 2%
◆ the probability of having a positive result with an amniocentesis (including both true positives and false positives) is 2.8%
◆ the probability of having a positive result with CVS (including both true positives and false positives) is 5.1%
◆ the probability of having a negative result with amniocentesis is 97.2%
◆ the probability of having a negative result with CVS is 94.9%
◆ the probability of having a false negative test result with amniocentesis is 0%
◆ the probability of having a false negative test result with CVS is 0.1%.

The probability of each set of branches in the decision model should always add up to 1 (remember, probability ranges from 0 being impossible though to 1.0 being certain, if all possible options are included in the tree

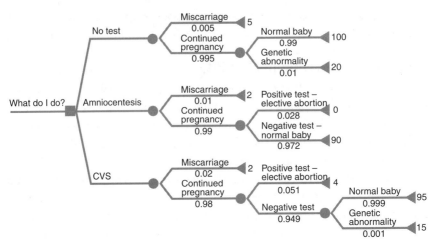

Figure 8.3 Prenatal testing decision with probability and utility values added.

then together they will sum to 1). The probability values have been added to the trees and are shown in Figure 8.3.

Step three – attach utilities/values to the tree

Utility measurement is a particular feature of decision analysis and is an attempt to attach a numerical value to the decision maker's views or feelings regarding the different decision tree outcomes. Conventionally, utilities are measured on a numerical scale with 0 representing the worst possible outcome (often death) and 100 representing the best possible outcome (often full health). Measuring utilities raises questions regarding whose utilities should be measured in a decision model and whether it is acceptable to use practitioners' or families' estimations of patient utility. Several studies highlight the possibility that patient utility for different outcomes can differ significantly from practitioner utility (Kramer et al., 1990). There is also some debate concerning whether individual utility assessments should be used, or calculations based on general societal evaluations (Chapman & Sonnenberg, 2000). We have assumed that utility values will be elicited from the individual involved in making the decision (be it patient or client).

An individual's utility can be measured in a variety of ways, each of which has benefits and limitations. One of the simplest ways of assessing utility is via rating scales. These consist of a line on a page, with clearly defined end points and interval markers. The decision maker is asked to place each of the health states in the decision model along the line to illustrate their differences in preference. However, these methods are not considered to be particularly useful because individuals tend to avoid the extremes in the scales (Thornton et al., 1992). Other methods of utility measurement include time trade off and standard gamble (lottery) techniques.

In time trade off the decision maker considers the relative amount of time they would be prepared to spend in a variety of health states (e.g. would you be prepared to trade 5 years of full health for 10 years with heart disease?).

In standard gamble techniques, the decision maker is asked to make a variety of choices between two decision alternatives: one with a certain outcome, the other being a gamble. The stage at which the person is no longer prepared to gamble provides the utility for that particular option (Drummond, 1993). For example, using the decision tree that we have already developed, you need to determine the woman's utility for having a baby with a genetic abnormality. You would give her a scenario where she has two options:

◆ option 1, where she takes a gamble that there is a 10% probability of having a miscarriage and the baby dying and a 90% chance that the baby will be normal
◆ option 2, which is the certain outcome that the baby will have a genetic abnormality.

The woman then has to say which option she would prefer. Depending on her answer you repeat the question, changing the probabilities for the gamble, until she is indifferent between the gamble and the certainty. The probability at this point is deemed to be equivalent to her utility for the health state (Drummond, 1993). In this instance, say at a 25% probability of miscarriage versus a 75% probability of a normal baby, the woman is indifferent between the two options. This means that her utility for having a baby with a genetic abnormality is 25.

A number of 'off the shelf' utility values can be used in decision analytic models. One of the most common is the QALY or quality adjusted life year. Sox et al. (1988, p. 217) define a QALY as 'the period of time in perfect health that a patient says is equivalent to a year in a state of ill health'. Unlike the individual measures of utility described above, QALYs are often values attached to different health states that have been calculated from general population data. A QALY is expressed in terms of the number of years in perfect health, reflecting the desirability of different outcomes with respect to quality and length of life (Stiggelbout, 2000). For example,

4 years in a health state that is valued at a quarter of perfect health (having a utility of 0.25) is equivalent to one QALY ($4 \times 0.25 = 1$).

For the sake of the example in Scenario 8.1, imagine that, having established the woman's utilities, you arrive at the following utility values with her:

◆ no test and miscarriage: 5
◆ no test and child with genetic abnormality: 20
◆ no test and normal baby: 100
◆ amniocentesis then miscarriage: 2
◆ amniocentesis, positive test, then elective abortion: 0
◆ amniocentesis, negative test, then normal baby: 90
◆ CVS then miscarriage: 2
◆ CVS, positive test, then elective abortion: 4
◆ CVS, negative test, then child with genetic abnormality: 15
◆ CVS, negative test, then normal baby: 95.

In this example, the woman attaches the highest utility of 100 (i.e. she highly values) to having a normal baby. It is also clear that there is some loss of utility associated with going through the anxiety of having an amniocentesis or CVS test (90 or 95, a 10 or 5 utility difference from the optimum). She feels having a positive test result after amniocentesis would be the worst possible outcome (0), followed by having the test then miscarrying (2). There is some utility attached to having a positive test and abortion earlier in her pregnancy with the CVS test, as opposed to amniocentesis (4 as opposed to 0). Having a baby with a genetic abnormality is slightly more positive than miscarrying (in the context of calculated utilities). Her values for the different outcomes have been added to the decision tree in Figure 8.3.

Utility elicitation is a highly individual process and each person will probably have different values for each of the different outcomes.

Step four – identify the option that maximises expected utility

The next step in the analysis is to calculate the decision tree. This is done by multiplying utility and probability values for each chance outcome, adding them up and then doing the same thing for each decision branch – again working from right to left. For example, the utility of not having a test and miscarrying (5) is multiplied by the probability of this occurring (0.005), which equals 0.025. The utility of not having a test and having a healthy baby is multiplied by the associated probability ($100 \times 0.99 = 99$) and added to the utility of not having a test and having a child with

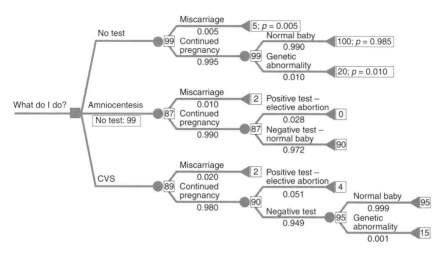

- **No test:** *Miscarriage* = 0.01 × 5 = 0.05.
  Continued pregnancy = ((0.99 × 100) + (0.01 × 20)) × 0.99 = (99 + 0.2) × 0.99 = 98.2.
  Expected utility for branch = 0.05 + 98.2 = **98.25**

- **Amniocentesis:** *Miscarriage* = 0.07 × 2 = 0.14.
  Continued pregnancy = ((0.028 × 0) + (0.972 × 90)) × 0.93 = (0 + 87.48) × 0.93 = 81.4.
  Expected utility for branch = 0.14 + 81.4 = **81.54**

- **CVS:** *Miscarriage* = 0.09 × 2 = 0.18.
  Continued pregnancy = ((0.051 × 4) + ((0.999 × 95) + (0.001 × 15) × 0.949) × 0.91 = (0.2 +
  ((94.9 + 0.015) × 0.949)) × 0.91 = (0.2 + 90.1) × 0.91 = **82.2**

Figure 8.4 Calculated prenatal testing decision tree.

a genetic abnormality (20 × 0.01 = 0.2 then 99 + 0.2 = 99.2). This is then multiplied by the probability of the pregnancy continuing (99.2 × 0.995 = 98.7). Finally the values for both sets of branches is summed (98.7 + 0.025 = 98.73) to provide the value for the 'no tests' branch (known as the expected value for that option). A similar calculation can be carried out for the 'have amniocentesis' branch, giving a sum of 87, and the 'have CVS' branch, giving a sum of 89 (the full tree, with calculations, is shown in Fig. 8.4).

As the model is rational, the option the woman should choose is not to have a test, because this is the option with the highest numerical value and therefore the one that maximises her expected utility – utilities that she helped establish.

Step five – carry out a sensitivity analysis

The results of any decision analysis model are dependent on the values built into the tree. A sensitivity analysis varies the probability and utility values within the tree systematically to identify threshold values: the points at which the optimum decision would change. This is particularly important if the probability values entered into the model are best estimates, rather than derived from research evidence, or there are very small differences in utility between the different outcomes.

A sensitivity analysis has been carried out on the example provided, varying the utility values for each outcome. This shows that the expected values of the branches are dependent on the utility values for one outcome: that of not having a test and having a normal baby. We can see that it is dependent, because varying the utility values for all of the other outcomes does not affect the decision result. This sensitivity analysis indicates that the woman's decision would alter if her utility value for not having a test and having a normal baby was 89.6 or lower. This means that if the woman's utility for having a normal baby without testing changed from 100 to 75, then the optimum decision for her would also change to having an amniocentesis or CVS test.

DECISION ANALYSIS AND CLINICAL DECISIONS: PRACTICAL EXAMPLES

As with many of the other concepts and decision aids discussed throughout this book, the majority of the research using decision analysis as an aid to decision making has been carried out in medicine, examining medical decisions. However, there are a few exceptions to this. For example, Lanza and Bantly (1991) used decision analytic techniques to examine the types of intervention that should be used for psychiatric patients assessed as having the potential for violence. They constructed the decision tree, identifying different possible interventions such as verbal interventions (for example, one to one meeting or community meeting) and physical interventions (for example, medication or a quiet room). The figures used in this particular decision model were estimates of probability and arbitrary values for utility measures. However, this tree has not been used in practice, so it is difficult to assess what impact it could have on practitioners.

Mosher et al. (1999) examined the usefulness of four different debridement agents for necrotic pressure sores. They constructed decision trees based on existing hospital protocols for the use of the different agents but were unable to identify any relevant research literature regarding outcomes of the agents (in terms of complete debridement and rates of infection).

After consulting experts in the field, they used delphi techniques to obtain consensus estimates of the probability for intervention outcomes. They chose not to measure patient utility in the model, instead examining utility in terms of monetary cost and nursing time associated with each treatment. The authors identified the collagenase debriding agents as being the most cost effective option for the patient scenario they had constructed.

Other studies have used systematic decision support tools and decision trees (not specifically based on decision analysis) and have found that they improve decision accuracy when used in practice (Letourneau & Jensen, 1998) and can have direct, and beneficial, effects on the quality of patient care as expressed by indicators such as incidence of pressure sores (Warren et al., 1999).

Decision analysis has also been used as a teaching aid. Shamian (1991) found that a group of students taught to use clinical decision analysis made significantly more 'correct' decisions (i.e. they concurred with a group of experts), than a control group. This study also suggests that decision analytic techniques can foster higher consistency between nurses regarding the choice of clinical interventions deployed for clinical problems.

As with any aid to judgement and decision making, decision analysis is not appropriate for all the kinds of decisions that nurses, midwives and health visitors make. For example, decision analytic techniques are suited to helping people select interventions and are not too amenable to examining the hermeneutic or experiential choices faced by nurses (see Ch. 6). However, for decisions where you do have time to contemplate different treatment options, where the decision is complex, the outcomes are uncertain and where the patient or client views are important, it could be a useful addition to a nurses' toolkit of techniques for aiding decision making.

Examples of practice where it could potentially be used include:

◆ decisions regarding what type of therapeutic mattress to use for a patient at risk of pressure sores
◆ decisions regarding what type of dressing to put on a chronically infected wound
◆ decisions regarding what type of pain therapy to use for chronically ill patients.

It is worth highlighting the potential role of decision analysis in providing counselling support and treatment advice to patients. The technique has the ability to display clearly the different options open to the patient or client, and allows the practitioner to fully explore the consequences of different options with them.

STRENGTHS AND WEAKNESSES OF DECISION ANALYSIS

As with all tools that intended to aid decision making and judgement, decision analysis has both strengths and weaknesses.

Letourneau and Jensen (1998) suggest that decision trees are useful in nursing practice because they help nurses to collect the most relevant information in particular clinical situations, as well as improving decision accuracy. As with judgement analytic approaches (see Ch. 5), the consistent and systematic approach provided by decision analysis can have a positive effect on the quality of care patients receive (Letourneau & Jensen, 1998).

Dowie (1996, p.17) proposes that the approach can fulfil a vital 'frame-working' role for policy development 'ensuring that all components in a decision are addressed systematically and explicitly in research and practice'.

Lanza and Bantly (1991) suggest that decision analysis is an efficient way of learning clinical problems because it forces a reasoned scientific and systematic approach to decision making, leading to efficiency. It also makes all of the assumptions taken within the decision problem explicit, clearly showing the decision processes used (Doubilet & McNeil, 1988).

With the policy imperative of clinical governance and evidence based practice, together with the growing emphasis on inclusive ways of involving patients in decision making processes, decision analysis also offers the ability to incorporate research evidence explicitly into decision situations. It clearly addresses the values of the individual making the decision (often the patient) and provides a record of how the decision was reached.

However, decision analysis is only as good as the assumptions that have been used to build the decision model (Mosher et al., 1999). There is always a danger that the tree structure may not be detailed enough to address the decision situation fully or be too detailed, and therefore too complicated, to use. Often the data needed to estimate probability accurately do not exist, which means that probability values are taken from subjective estimates. These subjective estimates of probability are prone to the types of bias that have been highlighted in Chapter 2. For instance the probability of a particular event occurring may be over estimated (over confidence) or under estimated because of the under confidence and over compensation of the expert. They may also use heuristics such as availability, representativeness or anchoring when estimating probability (Balla et al., 1989), all of which will affect the results of the model.

There are also problems with the estimation of utility itself. The type of method used to elicit utility values will invariably affect the result, as will the way different chance options are framed or put to the decision maker. There is also some concern regarding attaching numerical values to complex health situations at all 'To equate death with zero and amputation or hemiplegia with 0.3 or 0.4 appears to be an overprecise way of measuring something which may well be immeasurable.' (Balla et al., 1989). Issues also surround the validity of asking individuals to contemplate a decision to place a value on a situation for which they have no previous experience (for example, how do you really know what it is like to have a Down syndrome child, unless you have one?). Chapman and Sonnenberg (2000) highlight that patients who are contemplating a decision are more likely to place a negative estimate on predicted 'guestimates' of adverse effects from complications of treatment than they are after the treatment has been experienced.

However, responses to criticism of decision analysis highlight that any form of decision making is open to bias and limitations in available data. All decision analysis does is make those biases open to examination (Doubilet & McNeil, 1988).

CONCLUSION

Decision analysis is a powerful tool for use in certain clinical problems. As Lanza and Bantly (1991, p. 60) suggest 'Decision analysis makes explicit those often implicit considerations to assist nurses in making the best possible clinical choice in difficult or complex situations'.

Through explicitly structuring decision or treatment options with a patient or client, factoring in the probability of events occurring, and their own values or utility, a productive aid to clinical decision making can be generated. However, as with any clinical technique, you need to be aware of both its benefits and its limitations. You also need to be sure that it is an appropriate tool for the type of decision you need to make.

QUESTIONS FOR DISCUSSION

◆ What types of decisions do you make in practice that might be suitable for a decision analytic approach?

◆ Do you know what the research evidence is for the different choice and chance options within the decision?

◆ Do you explicitly take your patient/client values and beliefs about the different options into account when you make decisions?

ANNOTATED FURTHER READING

Decision analysis in nursing is an underused technique, so most texts are either psychological or medical in origin. The two books recommended consider issues regarding decision analysis in medicine in more detail than covered here.

Chapman, G.B. & Sonnenberg, F.A. (2000). *Decision making in health care. Theory, psychology and applications.* Cambridge: Cambridge University Press.

Llewelyn, H. & Hopkins, A. (1993). *Analysing how we reach clinical decisions.* London: Royal College of Physicians.

REFERENCES

Alfirevic, Z., Gosden, C.M., & Neilson, J.P. (2000). Chorion villus sampling versus amniocentesis for prenatal diagnosis (Cochrane Review). In: *The Cochrane Library*, issue 4. Oxford: Update Software.

Balla, J.I., Elstein, A., & Christensen, C. (1989). Obstacles to the acceptance of clinical decision analysis. *British Medical Journal, 298*, 579–582.

Chapman, G.B. & Sonnenberg, F.A. (2000). Introduction. In: Chapman, G.B. & Sonnenberg, F.A. (eds), *Decision making in health care. Theory, psychology and applications* (pp. 3–19). Cambridge: Cambridge University Press.

Doubilet, P. & McNeil, B.J. (1988). Clinical decision making. In: Dowie, J. & Elstein, A. (eds), *Professional judgment: A reader in clinical decision making* (pp. 255–276). Cambridge: Cambridge University Press.

Dowie, J. (1992). *Professional judgement and decision making. Introductory texts 5 to 7.* Milton Keynes: The Open University.

Dowie, J. (1996). The research–practice gap and the role of decision analysis in closing it. *Health Care Analysis, 4*, 5–18.

Drummond, M. (1993). Estimating utilities for making decisions in health care. In: Llewelyn, H. & Hopkins, A. (eds), *Analysing how we reach clinical decisions* (pp. 125–144). London: Royal College of Physicians of London.

Kramer, M.S., MacLellan, A.M., Ciampi, A., Etezadi-Amoli, J., & Leduc, D.G. (1990). Parents' vs physicians' utilities (values) for clinical outcomes in potentially bacteremic children. *Journal of Clinical Epidemiology, 43*(12), 1319–1325.

Lanza, M.L. & Bantly, A. (1991). Decision analysis: A method to improve quality of care for nursing practice. *Journal of Nursing Care and Quality, 6*(1), 60–72.

Letourneau, S. & Jensen, L. (1998). Impact of a decision tree on chronic wound care. *Journal of Wound, Ostomy and Continence Nursing, 25*, 240–247.

Llewelyn, H. & Hopkins, A. (1993). *Analysing how we reach clinical decisions.* London: Royal College of Physicians of London.

Mosher, B.A., Cuddigan, J., Thomas, D.R., & Boudreau, D.M. (1999). Outcomes of 4 methods of debridement using a decision analysis methodology. *Advances in Wound Care, 12*(Suppl 2), 12–21.

Panniers, T.L. & Walker, E.K. (1994). A decision-analytic approach to clinical nursing. *Nursing Research, 43*(4), 245–249.

Pauker, S.P. & Pauker, S.G. (1977). Prenatal diagnosis: A directive approach to genetic counselling using decision analysis. *The Yale Journal of Biology and Medicine, 50,* 275–289.

Shamian, J. (1991). Effect of teaching decision analysis on student nurses' clinical intervention decision making. *Research in Nursing and Health, 14,* 59–66.

Thornton, J.G., Lilford, R.J., & Johnson, N. (1992). Decision analysis in medicine. *British Medical Journal, 304,* 1099–1103.

Warren, J.B., Yoder, L.H., & Young-McCaughan, S. (1999). Development of a decision tree for support surfaces: A tool for nursing. *MedSurg Nursing, 8*(4), 239–248.

9

Clinical guidelines

Jo Rycroft-Malone

KEY ISSUES

◆ Clinical guidelines are at the heart of attempts to improve the quality of clinical decision making in health services.

◆ Guidelines have the power to reduce inappropriate variability in decision making and improve outcomes.

◆ Guidelines are not a panacea (or a replacement) for professional clinical decision making or judgement.

◆ Means of developing guidelines where little or no evidence exists need to be explored.

Clinical guidelines are at the heart of NHS quality improvement (DoH, 1997, 1998; Scottish Office, 1999; Welsh Office, 1998). The advent of clinical governance has increased interest in the evidence base for clinical decision making and effectiveness of care. The establishment of the National Institute for Clinical Excellence (NICE) and its ambitious programme of guideline development also signals a political and financial commitment to this important form of decision technology.

WHAT ARE CLINICAL GUIDELINES?

Clinical guidelines are 'systematically developed statements to assist practitioner and patient decisions about appropriate healthcare for specific circumstances' (Institute of Medicine, 1992). They are recommendations for the care of clients or patients with a particular condition, disease or set of symptoms. The amount of operational information within guidelines, and the degree to which a guideline is considered 'optional', varies. National clinical guidelines, interpreted and implemented locally, are sometimes referred to as protocols (Duff et al., 1996a).

It is tempting to accept guidelines at face value, particularly when recommendations are linked to professional organisations or government bodies. It is pertinent, therefore, to open this chapter by examining the contribution of guidelines to practice and by considering their potential benefits and limitations.

WHAT CONTRIBUTION DO CLINICAL GUIDELINES MAKE TO PRACTICE?

Potential benefits

The principal contribution of guidelines is an improvement in the quality of care received by patients. Guidelines are a mechanism for reducing inappropriate variations in clinical practice and discouraging practices that do not have convincing or sufficient evidence of effectiveness (Field & Lohr, 1990). Evaluations of clinical guidelines have demonstrated that improvements in the quality of care delivered in health services are possible (Grimshaw & Russell, 1993a). However, these effects are variable and the extent to which guidelines are implemented routinely in daily clinical practice is less clear (Thomas et al., 1999).

Decisions in health care involve weighing the potential benefits and harms of interventions whilst bearing in mind the impact of limited resources and populations with varying health care needs. Focusing on evidence based health care has led to the realisation that the task of accessing and interpreting 'raw' research evidence in everyday practice is nigh on impossible for most practitioners. Because of the volume of journals and articles available, the practical difficulties of accessing libraries and databases, and the need to acquire skills for determining the quality and validity of research, there is a clear need for synthesised evidence with explicit recommendations for practice. Guidelines help clinicians reduce the impact of selective memory recall and limited time for appraisal and synthesis of research. At the same time, guidelines foster an appreciation of the quality of knowledge derived by systematically reviewing available and appropriate research evidence.

Clinical guidelines contribute to the dissemination and implementation of evidence based practice in three ways (Rycroft-Malone & Duff, 2000):

◆ providing knowledge about care options that practitioners can draw on when making clinical decisions with patients
◆ outlining a course of treatment or interventions that can act as a blueprint for care. This is particularly useful in supporting quality improvement activities such as care pathways (Currie & Harvey, 2000)
◆ providing evidence-based definitions for care, against which practice, and sometimes costs, can be measured.

Guidelines offer benefits for the users of services. Woolf et al. (2000) argue that the greatest benefit is in improved health outcomes. Guidelines achieve this by recommending the most effective or beneficial practices and discouraging those that are ineffective or harmful. Guidelines specially adapted for users provide a resource or information guide to help them make informed choices and provide them with criteria against which to evaluate the appropriateness of the care they are offered.

Potential limitations

Guidelines can contribute to an illusion of a single answer for complex decision problems (Berg, 1997). Whilst guidelines should contain a synthesis of the best available research evidence, clinical decision making does not take place in a contextual 'vacuum'. When selecting the best treatment for patients, practitioners operate in a complex environment and whilst recommendations in guidelines are weighted according to the robustness of the evidence supporting them, their implementation is dependent upon agreement between both practitioner and patient. Clearly guidelines can never (and should not claim to) cover all the decisions that practitioners have to make in the 'swampy lowlands of [professional] practice' (Schon, 1991).

A further limitation of guidelines is that recommendations might simply be wrong. There are a number of desirable attributes for guidelines (Table 9.1), which if not addressed during the development process can

Table 9.1 Desirable attributes of clinical guidelines

Attribute	Meaning
Validity	Correctly interpreting available evidence so that implementation will yield health improvements
Cost effectiveness	Generating health improvements at acceptable cost
Reproducibility	On the same evidence, another group would have made the same recommendations
Reliability	In the same circumstances, another group of health professionals would apply the guidelines similarly
Representative	All key disciplines and interests (including patients) contributed to the development of the guidelines
Clinical applicability	Target population defined in accordance with the evidence
Clinical flexibility	Exceptions are identified, as are patient preferences
Clarity	Precise, unambiguous and user friendly
Meticulous	Recording of participants, documentation assumptions and methods
Scheduled review	When and how they will be reviewed
Utilisation review	Indications of ways in which adherence may be monitored

result in flawed recommendations – with the potentially harmful effects for patients that such flaws imply.

Additionally, only a small amount of what health care practitioners do and, in particular, what nurses do, is represented in well designed and conducted studies. Those studies that exist are often flawed and poorly reported, leading to bias and misleading findings. In such cases, and in the absence of time and skills to scrutinise every piece of available research, value judgements made by guideline development groups may represent the wrong choices for individual patients (Woolf et al., 2000).

Given the apparently mixed contribution that guidelines can make to patient care, the reader would be right to conclude that such technologies are no panacea for achieving evidence based practice. However, they do have a role to play in integrating research evidence into clinical decision making and thus improving the quality of care delivered by nurses. The remainder of the chapter explores the guideline development process and considers the relative strengths and weaknesses of the various techniques employed. In doing so, the chapter draws on examples from the national guideline development completed under the auspices of the Royal College of Nursing Institute.

HOW ARE CLINICAL GUIDELINES DEVELOPED?

The nature of 'evidence'

Clearly, a key defining attribute of a clinical guideline is that recommendations are based on evidence. Definitions of evidence based practice recognise that blanket application of research evidence are inadequate (Kitson et al., 1998). Practitioners must recognise that the best care depends not only on identifying the best care for populations of patients (from appropriate research evidence), but also on ascertaining the most appropriate care for meeting the identified needs of particular individuals. It is in making this judgement that clinical expertise adds a third component to the evidence base for making decisions. Therefore, clinically effective care needs due weight to be attached to:

◆ knowledge from research findings
◆ knowledge from clinical experience (expertise)
◆ patient specific information: including the preferences and the acceptability of an intervention to an individual patient.

These same sources of 'evidence' can be used to inform the development of clinical guidelines.

Guideline development group

Clinical guidelines can be produced nationally or locally and are usually written by a group. The composition of a guideline development group is an important component in the eventual validity and acceptability of the resultant guideline (Duff et al., 1996a). To ensure that all aspects of a condition, care or intervention are addressed it is important that the group is multidisciplinary (Leape et al., 1992). Lomas (1993) outlines three reasons why this representation is important:

◆ the limited information available for guideline developers needs to be supplemented by the interpretations of these stakeholders
◆ legitimate conflicts over values need to be resolved
◆ the successful introduction of a guideline requires that all key disciplines contribute to its development to ensure ownership and support.

Patients, clients or their representatives should also be included in guideline development. Their participation ensures that users are more actively involved in deciding what they consider to be effective care and adds another dimension to descriptions of clinically effective care (Duff et al., 1996b).

Guideline development methods

The quality of the guideline development process is important because it influences the credibility of the guideline as well as its validity. Woolf (1992) describes three broad methods of guideline development – adding that these are by no means mutually exclusive:

◆ evidence linked guideline development
◆ informal consensus approaches
◆ formal consensus methods.

Evidence linked guideline development Recommendations are based on a systematic review of the literature and make explicit linkage to the level of supporting evidence. This linkage enables clinicians to make decisions about levels of adherence to the guideline. Grimshaw et al. (1995) argue that, in cases where there is a strong level of supporting evidence, clinicians should have very good reasons for choosing not to comply. However, as Woolf (1992) states, whilst this approach can be credited with enhancing the scientific rigour of guidelines, in the absence of acceptable evidence one is unable to produce recommendations.

Informal consensus approaches Woolf (1992) suggests that this is the most common method of guideline development. This method is most frequently used at a local level where committees formulate recommendations without drawing on research evidence (Grimshaw & Hutchinson, 1995). By definition, this method tends to be based on poorly defined criteria, often lacking explicit statements of consensus; consequently, resulting guidelines tend to be subjective and ill defined.

Formal consensus methods Methods such as Delphi or Nominal Group Technique provide a structure for the group decision making process by, for example, adopting rating methods to represent the extent of agreement regarding predefined issues or questions. However, they are criticised for: (i) being opaque to external observers (Grimshaw & Hutchinson, 1995); and (ii) not providing an explicit linkage between recommendations and the quality of evidence (Grimshaw et al., 1995; Woolf, 1992).

Ideally, guideline development should be based on high quality research evidence, which is appropriately matched to the question(s) asked. In situations where there is little good quality evidence, guideline developers need to adopt alternative strategies – or not develop the guideline until a suitable body of evidence becomes available. Given the need for clinicians to make decisions in situations where the evidence base has not been determined (Eccles et al., 1996) developing guidelines based on a framework that utilises facets of more than one guideline development method seems appropriate. However, in doing so developers need to be transparent regarding the process they adopt and explicitly link recommendations to the evidence source(s) they draw on.

Guideline development based on systematic review

Broadly, the most important steps in the development of a guideline can be summarised as:

◆ basing the recommendations on the best evidence available (Woolf, 1996) – generally these will be derived from a systematic review of published and unpublished literature (Mulrow & Oxman, 1996; NHS Centre for Reviews and Dissemination (CRD), 1996)
◆ making an explicit linkage between guideline recommendations and the quality of the evidence underpinning them
◆ utilising the skills of a multidisciplinary group, including user representatives. The group should have clinical or research experience in the areas addressed by the guideline.

Figure 9.1 identifies the steps taken in the development of a guideline for the management of patients with venous leg ulcers (Royal College of Nursing Institute et al., 1998). In this example, the guideline group accessed a wide research base and looked at a number of well conducted systematic reviews of research literature. This method was developed based on the methodology of other guideline developers (Deighan, 1993; Eccles et al., 1996; Royal College of Psychiatrists, 1997; Waddell et al., 1996; Woolf, 1992) and the appraisal criteria outlined in Table 9.1.

- Topic of guideline determined by review group and availability of research evidence
  - Develop evidence model to clarify the scope of the guideline
    - Inclusion/exclusion criteria for evidence identified
    - Literature searches conducted using selection criteria
(computerised databases, hand searching, grey literature, expert contacts, industry)
    - Abstracts sifted for fulfilment of criteria and clinical relevance
      - Full copies of pertinent articles requested
  - Each article appraised by two reviewers for validity and relevance
    - Data extracted using standardised forms by the two reviewers
  - Data extraction forms, quality checklists and articles returned to the guideline developer
    - Every fifth article checked for quality of appraisal
- Arbitration for inconsistent conclusions about rejection or acceptance of findings provided by systematic review and topic expert(s)
  - Evidence from research literature synthesised by guideline developer
    - Guideline development group members read and critique review
  - Recommendations developed and graded by strength of underpinning evidence
  - Recommendations reviewed by review group, patient/carer group, external peer review group (all provided with summary of evidence)
- Clinical guidelines piloted for applicability, user-friendliness and comprehensiveness
      - Clinical guideline revised
    - Guideline produced as Full Recommendations, Summary Version, Technical Report and Implementation Guide
      - Dissemination

Figure 9.1 Guideline development process for the management of patients with venous leg ulcers. Reproduced with permission from Royal College of Nursing (1998).

This process illustrates the steps required to perform a systematic review through to guideline dissemination. The purpose of doing a systematic review is to collect all the research evidence, assess its potential applicability to the clinical topic of the guideline, critically appraise the evidence for bias and extract and summarise the findings. Adhering to the standards of guideline development can be a lengthy process.

It is worth highlighting that whilst this guideline development method constitutes best practice – because it increases the validity of a guideline – it is not immune to the effects of bias. A stepwise and logical process has been illustrated, with every stage representing a decision making point for the developer and development group. Critical appraisal choices, inclusion and exclusion of research, and the interpretation of research, can be subject to an individual's biases. It is therefore vital that the processes used to make decisions are transparent so that guideline users can make their own judgements on the validity of the end product.

One of the advantages of being able to develop a guideline from a systematic review is that it is easier to formulate brief and unequivocal recommendations if they are founded on well conducted studies (McInnes et al., 2000). The consequence being that if recommendations are implemented improvements in care and outcomes are more likely. The grading of recommendations (see Table 9.2 for an example) gives guideline users an indication of the strength of the evidence underpinning them. However, even with grade I recommendations, implementation requires a degree of interpretation on the part of the clinician. An example of this can be found

Table 9.2 Grading system. Adapted from Waddell et al. (1996)

Grade (strength of recommendation)	Criteria
I	Generally consistent finding in a majority of multiple *acceptable* studies
II	Either based on a single *acceptable* study or on a weak or inconsistent finding in multiple *acceptable* studies
III	Limited scientific evidence that does not meet all the criteria of *acceptable* studies or absence of directly applicable studies of good quality. This includes expert opinion

Acceptable *refers to studies that have been subjected and approved by a process of critical appraisal.*

in the guideline *The management of venous leg ulcers* (Royal College of Nursing Institute et al., 1998).

In this guideline the supporting evidence for the application of multi-layered high compression bandaging for uncomplicated leg ulcers is strong and convincing and thus this recommendation is graded as I. However, the evidence does not enable a recommendation to be made about the number of bandaging layers and is therefore open to practitioner interpretation in conjunction with patient wishes. This highlights the challenge practitioners face when trying to balance various different types of evidence in the clinical decision making process.

Guideline development when the evidence base is weak

Whilst the most valid guidelines tend to be defined by the quality of the research evidence available, many aspects of health care do not have a good research knowledge base. Purists would argue that in such cases guidelines should not be developed. Realists would counter with an acknowledgement that nurses constantly make decisions for which there is no research evidence base. To exclude recommendations on the basis of no (or weak) research evidence would result in a guideline of only limited utility for clinicians. Whilst authors such as Grimshaw and Russell (1993b) and Shekelle et al. (1999) acknowledge the use of opinion to formulate recommendations, they rightly point out that the process adopted has to be explicit and the source material for recommendations in the resultant guideline clearly documented. If guidelines do incorporate expert opinion this must be gathered in a systematic way and the use of formal consensus processes are recommended.

Figure 9.2 represents the steps taken in the formal consensus process adopted in the development of the guideline *Pressure ulcer risk assessment and prevention* (Royal College of Nursing Institute, 2000), which advanced the use of consensus methods in national guideline development in the UK (NICE Clinical Guidelines Advisory Committee, 2000). It achieved this because it systematically, comprehensively and explicitly sought the opinion of experts. This was in opposition to the traditional *ad hoc* and unsystematic technique of informal consensus or GOBSAT (good old boys sitting around the table chatting!).

This guideline could draw on two pertinent systematic reviews, but their clinical scope was limited. Consequently, it was necessary to develop a guideline that contained a mixture of evidence based and consensus based recommendations. A more detailed account of the method can be found elsewhere (Rycroft-Malone, 2000).

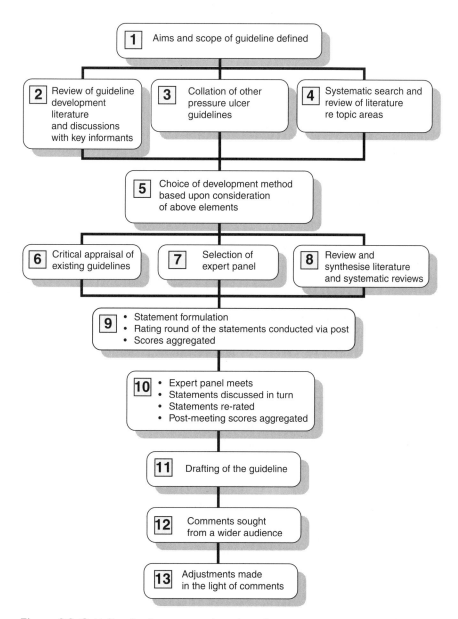

Figure 9.2 Guideline development – using a formal consensus process.

Clearly, however, the use of opinion in guideline development has its limitations 'clinical guidelines are valid if, when followed, they lead to the health gains and costs predicted for them' (Grimshaw & Russell, 1993b, p. 245).

Ensuring validity

The validity of a guideline resulting from a process such as the one outlined in Figure 9.2 is open to question. Grimshaw and Russell (1993b) argue that validity is dependent upon:

◆ how the evidence was identified and synthesised
◆ how many guideline users and key disciplines were included in the guideline group
◆ the way the guideline was developed.

Based on these criteria, guidelines with greater scientific validity will be those that:

◆ are developed from systematic reviews
◆ include most key disciplines
◆ ensure the explicit linkage of recommendations with evidence.

Guidelines developed with evidence derived from systematic reviews, as well as consensus opinion not entirely based on research evidence, would by the same criteria be viewed as less scientifically valid (Grimshaw & Hutchinson, 1995).

Given the basic premise that limiting recommendations to where evidence exists 'reduce[s] the scope of the guidelines and limit[s] their value to clinicians and policy makers who need to make decisions in the presence of imperfect knowledge' (Eccles et al., 1996, p. 47), perhaps the best we can do is try and identify a method that will produce more 'good' judgements than other methods (Murphy et al., 1998). This begs the questions: 'what method ensures arrival at good judgements?' and 'what is a good judgement?'.

Murphy et al. (1998) suggest that a good judgement is a valid judgement. They propose a number of ways to assess validity in consensus based guideline development processes, including predictive and concurrent validity and internal logic. For example, if validity is assessed concurrently it would mean that group decisions that conflict with research evidence without good reason would be invalid. However, there is no absolute means by which to judge whether (at the time) a decision was valid, and thus no means to assess the validity of the method via which it was made (Murphy et al., 1998). The recommendations could be assessed prospectively by, for example, an audit of guideline implementation.

Despite these weaknesses, there are some strengths associated with this guideline development process. Firstly, it provides an opportunity for collaborative working between a number of different disciplines at all stages of the development process. Secondly, and equally as important, this method provides a forum for patient and/or carer participation. This can be particularly useful in situations where little research about patient/carers' experiences of certain conditions and/or care exists. Finally, using a multi-professional, collaborative approach can enhance the credibility of the guideline to end users. That is, if the participants involved in the development process are recognised professionals in the particular field of practice, this can exert a positive influence on the uptake of the resulting guideline.

Guideline development – summary

The method of guideline development depends upon the:

◆ topic
◆ experience of the guideline development group
◆ purpose of the guideline and the evidence available (Thompson et al., 1999).

The most scientifically valid guidelines are those based on robust research evidence. In cases where there is not a good research base, systematic methods of gathering expert opinion must be employed to maximise guideline validity. Whether research or expert opinion forms the basis for the guideline, users should appraise the validity of a guideline before adopting it. Within the UK a number of tools have been developed that can assist individuals in this task (Cluzeau et al., 1997; Scottish Intercollegiate Guidelines Network, 1995).

GUIDELINE IMPLEMENTATION – LOCAL ADAPTATION

Clinical contexts for decision making are messy and complex. It would be naïve to suggest that the production and dissemination of a guideline automatically leads to changes in practice. Experience and research have demonstrated that successful implementation of guidelines is dependent upon a number of key elements, a particularly important one being a sense of ownership of the guideline amongst those charged with implementing it (Duff et al., 1996a).

Theories of change (Klein, 1976) and the findings of research in the field of quality improvement (Harvey, 1993; Kitson et al., 1994) demonstrate that professionals will oppose changes that they feel are a threat to their competence and autonomy. They might also distrust or disagree with guidelines written by national experts and instead rely on their own experience or the recommendations of their colleagues. Given that most organisations do not have adequate resources or skills to develop valid guidelines, the more favourable (and practical) option might be to adapt a national guideline for local use. This process also helps to overcome some of the likely barriers to change. Adaptation is a process that involves local clinicians, thus encouraging ownership leading to an increased likelihood of guideline uptake in practice. See *Implementing Clinical Guidelines* (The Clinical Guidelines Education Team, 2001) for details of how to adapt guidelines for local use.

CONCLUSION

The role of clinical guidelines as a tool for aiding decision making is gaining momentum. This renewed prominence is set against the background of the drive to improve the quality of care for patients and increase clinical effectiveness. There is also a steadily increasing body of evidence that guidelines can lead to improvements in both the process and outcomes of care (Dobson et al., 1999; Dunning et al., 1999; McLaren & Ross, 2000; NHS CRD & Nuffield Institute for Health, 1994; NHS CRD, 1999). There is no doubt that guidelines are of potential use to nurses because they synthesise evidence into clear recommendations for practice and thereby help to overcome some of the practical difficulties faced by practitioners in clinical areas. Perhaps another, as yet under utilised, use of guidelines is in encouraging and helping patients and carers to participate in decision making processes.

This chapter has highlighted the challenges associated with developing clinically valid guidelines. Only valid guidelines (if implemented) will improve the quality of care patients receive. As methods of guideline development and implementation evolve, we can look forward to better quality clinical guidelines and improved care.

Evidence based practice and professional judgement are not mutually exclusive, however, we are only just now beginning to understand how nurses make decisions and how different types of knowledge are utilised in these processes. The research knowledge base underpinning practice can be enhanced by scientifically valid, user friendly guideline recommendations, but only if nurses value them as a knowledge source, are able to access them and able to develop appropriate implementation strategies.

QUESTIONS FOR DISCUSSION

◆ Consider the sort of topics and practice issues that arise in your clinical area that might benefit from recommendations in the form of a clinical guideline.

- Think about the sort of evidence base this topic(s) has – if you had to develop the clinical guideline yourself, what method would you have to use?

- How would you ensure that the desirable attributes of clinical guidelines (see Table 9.1) are met?

- What sort of representation might you have on the guideline development group?

- How would you involve users in the process?

- Consider the ways in which such a guideline might help in clinical decision making.

- How would you 'sell' such as guideline to your colleagues?

ANNOTATED FURTHER READING

Hutchinson, A. & Baker, R. (1999). *Making use of guidelines in clinical practice.* Oxford: Radcliffe Medical Press.

Twelve edited chapters in which guideline development, appraisal, dissemination and implementation are explored.

National Institute for Clinical Excellence (http://www.nice.org.uk).

For information on completed and ongoing guideline development in the UK.

RCN Information Service Quality Improvement Programme (0207 647 3829/3830 or email: qiprogramme@rcn.org.uk).

For assistance and information on where to locate clinical guidelines.

Scottish Intercollegiate Guidelines Network (SIGN) (http://www.sign.ac.uk).

Develops and publishes guidelines. The full text of many of these is available from the website.

REFERENCES

Berg, M. (1997). Problems and promises of the protocol. *Social Science and Medicine, 44,* 1081–1088.

Cluzeau, F., Littlejohns, P., Grimshaw, J., & Feder, G. (1997). *Appraisal instrument for clinical guidelines.* London: St George's Hospital Medical School.

Currie, V.L. & Harvey, G. (2000). The use of care pathways as tools to support the implementation of evidence-based practice. *Journal of Interprofessional Care, 14*(4), 311–324.

Deighan, M. (1993). *Consensus strategy for mainly nursing led major clinical guidelines. Letter inviting tender.* Manchester: Health Services Management Unit, University of Manchester.

Department of Health (1997). *The New NHS: modern dependable.* London: The Stationery Office.

Department of Health (1998). *A first class service.* London: The Stationery Office.

Dobson, S., Gabbay, J., Locock, L., & Chambers, D. (1999). *Evaluation of PACE programme: Final report.* Templeton College, UK.

Duff, L.A., Kitson, A.L., Seers, K., & Humphris, D. (1996a). Clinical guidelines: An introduction to their development and implementation. *Journal of Advanced Nursing, 23,* 887–895.

Duff, L.A., Kelson, M., Marriot, S. et al. (1996b) Clinical guidelines: Involving patients and users of services. *Journal of Clinical Effectiveness, 1*(3), 104–112.

Dunning, M., Abi-Aad, G., Gilbert, D., Hutton, H., & Brown, C. (1999). *Experience, evidence and everyday practice. Creating systems for delivering effective health care.* London: Kings Fund.

Eccles, M., Clapp, Z., Grimshaw, J. et al. (1996). Developing valid guidelines: Methodological and procedural issues from the North of England Evidence Based Guideline Development Project. *Quality in Health Care, 5,* 44–50.

Field, M.J. & Lohr, K.N. (1990). *Clinical practice guidelines: Directions for a new program.* Washington: National Academy Press.

Grimshaw, J.M., Eccles, M. et al. (1995). Developing scientifically valid practice guidelines. *Journal of Evaluation in Clinical Practice, 1*(1), 37–48.

Grimshaw, J.M. & Hutchinson, A. (1995). Clinical practice guidelines – do they enhance value for money in health care? *British Medical Bulletin, 51*(4), 927–940.

Grimshaw, J.M. & Russell, I.T. (1993a). Effect of clinical guidelines on medical practice: A systematic review of rigorous evaluations. *Lancet, 342,* 1317–1322.

Grimshaw, J.M. & Russell, I.T. (1993b). Achieving health gains through clinical guidelines: I developing scientifically valid guidelines. *Quality Assurance in Health Care, 2,* 243–248.

Harvey, G. (1993). *Nursing quality: An evaluation of the key factors in the implementation process.* London: South Bank University.

Institute of Medicine (1992). *Guidelines for clinical practice: From development to use.* Washington: National Academy Press.

Kitson, A.L., Harvey, G., Hyndman, S., Sindhu, F., & Yerrell, P.H. (1994). *The impact of a nursing quality assurance approach, the Dynamic Standard Setting System (DySSSy) on Nursing Practice and Patient Outcomes (the ODySSSy project).* Oxford: National Institute for Nursing.

Klein, D. (1976). Some notes on the dynamic of resistance to change: The defender role. In: Bennis, W.G., Benne, K.D., Chin, R., & Corey, K.E. (eds), *The planning of change,* 3rd edn (pp. 117–124). New York: Holt, Rienhart & Winston.

Leape, L.L., Park, R.E., Kahan, J.P., & Brook, R.H. (1992). Group judgements of appropriateness: The effect of panel composition. *Quality Assurance in Health Care, 4,* 151–159.

Lomas, J. (1993). Making clinical policy explicit: Legislative policy making and lessons for developing practice guidelines. *International Journal of Technology Assessment in Health Care, 9,* 11–25.

McInnes, E., Cullum, N., Nelson, E.A., Luker, K., & Duff, L.A. (2000). The development of a national guideline on the management of venous leg ulcers. *Journal of Clinical Nursing, 9,* 208–217.

McLaren, S.M.G. & Ross, F. (2000). Implementation of evidence into practice settings: Some methodological issues arising from the South Thames Evidence Based Practice Project. *Clinical Effectiveness in Nursing, 4,* 99–108.

Mulrow, C. & Oxman, A. (eds) Cochrane Collaboration Handbook (1996). Version 3. Cochrane Library. Oxford: *Update Software.*

Murphy, M.K., Black, N., Lamping, D.L. et al. (1998). Consensus development methods and their use in clinical guideline development. *Health Technology Assessment, 2*(3).

NHS Centre for Reviews and Dissemination (1996). *Undertaking systematic reviews of research on effectiveness. CRD Report 4.* York: University of York.

NHS Centre for Reviews and Dissemination (1999). Getting evidence into practice. *Effective Health Care, 5,* 1–16.

NHS Centre for Reviews and Dissemination and Nuffield Institute for Health (1994). Implementing clinical practice guidelines: Can guidelines be used to improve clinical practice? *Effective Health Care,* 1–12.

NICE Clinical Guidelines Advisory Committee (2000). *Critical appraisal of pressure ulcer risk assessment and prevention guidelines.* London: NICE.

Royal College of Nursing Institute (2000). *Pressure ulcer risk assessment and prevention.* RCN Technical Report website (http://www.rcn.org.uk).

Royal College of Nursing Institute, Centre for Evidence-Based Nursing (University of York), & the School of Nursing, Midwifery and Health Visiting (University of Manchester) (1998). *The management of patients with venous leg ulcers.* London: RCN Publishing.

Royal College of Psychiatrists (1997). The management of violence in clinical settings: An evidence based guide. London: Royal College of Psychiatrists.

Rycroft-Malone, J. (2000). The challenge of a weak evidence base: Formal consensus and guideline development. *Journal of Clinical Excellence, 2,* 35–41.

Rycroft-Malone, J. & Duff, L.A. (2000). Developing clinical guidelines: Issues and challenges. *Journal of Tissue Viability, 10*(4), 144–153.

Schon, D. (1991). *The reflective practitioner,* 2nd edn. New York: Basic Books.

Scottish Intercollegiate Guidelines Network (SIGN) (1995). *Clinical guidelines criteria for appraisal for national use.* Edinburgh: The Network.

Scottish Office (1999). *Designed to care: Renewing the National Health Service in Scotland.* Edinburgh: Scottish Office.

Shekelle, P.G., Woolf S.H., Eccles, M., & Grimshaw, J. (1999). Developing guidelines. *British Medical Journal, 318*(27 February), 593–596.

The Clinical Guidelines Education Team (2001). *Implementing Clinical Guidelines: A Resource for the Healthcare Team.* London: Bailliere Tindall.

Thomas, L.H., McColl, E., Cullum, N., Rousseau, N., & Soutter, J. (1999). Clinical guidelines in nursing, midwifery and the therapies: A systematic review. *Journal of Advanced Nursing, 30*(1), 40–50.

Waddell, G., Feder, G., McIntosh, A., Lewis, M., & Hutchinson, A. (1996). *Low back pain evidence review.* London: Royal College of Practitioners.

Welsh Office (1998). *Putting patients first: Quality care and clinical excellence.* Cardiff: Welsh Office.

Woolf, S.H. (1992). Practice guidelines – a new reality in medicine II. Methods of developing guidelines. *Archives of Internal Medicine, 152,* 946–952.

Woolf, S.H. (1996). Developing evidence-based clinical practice guidelines. *Annual Review of Public Health, 17,* 511–538.

Woolf, S., Grol, R., Hutchinson, A., Eccles, M., & Grimshaw, J. (2000). The potential benefits, limitations and harms of clinical guidelines. In: Eccles, M. & Grimshaw, J. (eds), *Clinical guidelines from conception to use* (pp. 19–29). Oxford: Radcliffe Medical Press.

10

Computerised decision support

Robert Crouch

KEY ISSUES

◆ The quality and accuracy of assessment, judgement and decision making in clinical practice merits examination.

◆ Many opportunities for computerised decision support exist.

◆ Clinical decision making can be enhanced through the provision of decision support.

◆ Careful consideration should be given to the type and application of computerised decision support used in practice.

As already highlighted in previous chapters, nurses routinely conduct assessments and make judgements and decisions about patient management in clinical practice. However, those assessments, judgements and decisions are sometimes not as informed and accurate as they could be. The concept of computerised decision support as a way of aiding nurses' assessments, judgements and decisions is outlined in this chapter, together with discussion of the different approaches to designing and developing such technologies. An illustration from one area of practice – telephone consultation – is used to demonstrate potential benefits. The chapter concludes with a vision of the future of computer based decision support.

DECISION SUPPORT SOFTWARE: AN OVERVIEW

The term 'decision support software' encompasses any computer program designed to assist in professional clinical decision making (Shortliffe, 1990). Possible applications for such systems are numerous in both medicine and nursing. Early decision support applications included the generation of differential diagnosis in acute abdominal pain (de Dombal et al., 1972) and MYCIN, an expert system developed to provide assistance with the selection of antibiotic therapies (Shortliffe, 1976). Other applications are highlighted in Box 10.1.

Clearly, there is a broad range of applications for decision support software, and there is an equally broad range of theories and approaches underpinning these systems. The theoretical approach taken, and the level of decision support offered, are often determined by the end goal of the system; in health care these end goals include diagnosis, treatment and management.

Box 10.1 Applications for computerised decision support

◆ A system for assessing the aetiology of community acquired pneumonia (PNEUMON-IA; Verdaguer et al., 1992).

◆ Formulary decision making (RXPERT; Greer, 1992).

◆ Differential diagnosis of psychotic, mood and organic mental disorders (Monreno & Plant, 1993).

◆ Troubleshooting pulmonary artery catheter waveforms (Zielstorff et al., 1994).

◆ Teaching nursing diagnosis (Koch & McGovern, 1993).

◆ Computer assisted learning in renal nursing (Luker & Caress, 1992).

◆ Telephone consultation (Crouch et al., 1996a).

Dowie (1993) argues that the form of decision support that has been accepted best by clinicians is knowledge based. These technologies take the form of algorithms, flow diagrams or expert systems. These decision aids draw on the facts and assumptions about structures or processes that clinicians use to achieve best clinical practice. The internal reasoning is often based on cause–effect or 'if–then' type design rules (Dowie, 1993). An example would be the use of artificial intelligence (AI) models based on symbolic representations that are non-algorithmic (Clancey & Shortliffe, 1984). For medicine it is argued that a non-mathematical, or qualitative, approach is required; one that uses a variety of ways to problem solve. Buchanan and Shortliffe (1985) argue that problem solving approaches themselves are usually qualitative data reasoning techniques utilising judgement rules or heuristics, as well as theoretical laws and definitions. An example of an AI expert system is MYCIN (Duda & Shortliffe, 1983). MYCIN is designed to provide expert level solutions to a clinical problem. The system provides the rationale for the solution offered and is sufficiently flexible to accommodate new knowledge. Two elements are essential for such a system: a knowledge base and an inference engine.

The other type of decision aid is database oriented. Decisions are based on statistical inference rather than causal reasoning. For example, the decision aid used to generate the probability of someone presenting with a particular pattern of signs and symptoms of having a particular abdominal pathology uses a Bayesian approach, offering odds and guidance rather than specific conclusions (de Dombal, 1988; Dowie & Elstein, 1988).

Although many decision support systems have been developed, few are used routinely in clinical practice (Fox, 1993; Heathfield & Wyatt, 1993). There are several reasons given for this lack of uptake. Historically, the problems associated with technology, for example, the speed of computer processing, have been blamed. Also, the perception by users that there is limited (or no) use for the system (Heathfield & Wyatt, 1993); that they are too cumbersome to use in clinical practice (Wyatt & Spiegelhalter, 1990); and, lastly, that the focus of developers has often been the evaluation of a theoretical model (Heathfield & Wyatt, 1993). Heathfield and Wyatt (1993) argue that there is a need to build a coherent philosophy into all aspects of decision support software design and development, from inception of the idea to evaluation, maintenance and support. There are many applications for decision support software of differing degrees of complexity, together with different ways in which these systems can be classified.

CLASSIFICATION OF DECISION SUPPORT SOFTWARE

Shortliffe (1990) adopts a functionalist (i.e. what does it do?) stance in identifying three different ways that software can be used as a clinical tool (Box 10.2). Another method of classification is according to the clinical role performed by the software (Wyatt, 1991) (Box 10.3). The different types of systems described are not mutually exclusive; many decision support systems encompass two or more elements of each type.

Box 10.2 Classification of computerised decision support software by function (Shortliffe, 1990)

◆ *Information management* – this would include hospital information systems that contain patient specific data as well as those that store clinical information.

◆ *Focusing attention* – designed to remind clinicians of problems or diagnoses that might be overlooked.

◆ *Patient specific consultations* – these systems can provide therapeutic advice or diagnostic assistance. They use patient specific information or data to produce custom made information or advice about management. Statistical methods or simple logic may be employed in the problem solving. This last group are often called 'expert' systems.

◆ Interpreting patient data by sounding an alarm or highlighting an abnormal result.

◆ Requesting the user to input patient data and proposing a diagnosis or management plan.

◆ Allowing for flexible interaction and model building for joint negotiation of solutions.

DO WE NEED DECISION SUPPORT SOFTWARE?

As already stated at the beginning of this chapter, nurses routinely assess patients, make judgements about conditions and situations, and make decisions about plans of action or interventions. But how thorough are the assessments and how accurate are the judgements or decisions made? One area of practice where we have some insight into the answers to these questions is telephone consultation.

There have been a number of studies exploring the accuracy and adequacy of assessments made during telephone consultation both in primary care settings and in Emergency departments. The estimation of the adequacy and appropriateness of the assessments made range from 50% (Brown & Eberle, 1974) to 74% (Evans et al., 1993) of the calls reported. Inadequacies in the assessment of callers are highlighted by several studies. Aitken et al. (1995) found that inadequate advice was given in 16 out of 36 calls and was often based on very little information about the patient. In one case just the age of the infant was asked before the caller was advised to manage the problem at home. Inadequacies were also identified with a simulation of a patient with myocardial ischaemia, when 56% of nurses failed to ask any questions about the caller or the presenting complaint; only 9% of the callers were advised to call the emergency services (Verdile et al., 1989).

Variation in the adequacy of assessment has been identified across a number of presenting adult and paediatric complaints, and in a range of presenting problems from fever to chest pain (Brown & Eberle, 1974; Ott et al., 1974; Perrin & Goodman, 1978; Yanovski et al., 1992). A difference in the depth of assessment has been noted between nurses and other professional groups (Brown & Eberle, 1974; Evans et al., 1993; Isaacman et al., 1992; Perrin & Goodman, 1978; Sloane et al., 1985; Yanovski et al., 1992). Differences were identified between junior and experienced physicians, with experience proving beneficial in assessment and decision making (Sloane et al., 1985). One study in relation to paediatrics found nurse practitioner performance during telephone consultation was more effective in terms of patient assessment, history taking and disposition than experienced paediatricians and house officers (Perrin & Goodman, 1978).

In several studies, differences in consultation style, content and length were identified between clinicians with varying levels of experience and the assessment and advice given to the caller (Brown & Eberle, 1974; Greitzer et al., 1976; Isaacman et al., 1992; Ott et al., 1974; Perrin & Goodman, 1978; Sloane et al., 1985). Perrin and Goodman (1978) highlight the 'mind snapping shut' phenomenon, where the professional decides what is wrong with the patient and the most appropriate management plan too early in the patient encounter, sometimes before any history has been obtained beyond the presenting complaint. Yanovski et al. (1992) sought to establish whether experienced physicians (when compared with less experienced physicians) demonstrated superior telephone triage skills; they found no relationship between either the quantity or quality of questions asked and the length of experience.

Earlier studies, however, suggest that increasing experience is related to less time asking redundant questions, a lower number of questions asked during the assessment or problem solving part of the call and greater time spent on management aspects (Greitzer et al., 1976; Perrin & Goodman, 1978; Sloane et al., 1985). Whilst there is no evidence that deficiencies identified in assessment are rectified by experience or training (Brown & Eberle, 1974; Greitzer et al., 1976; Ott et al., 1974), the indicators of 'good' decision making used in these studies (the validity of the approaches used and the notion of decision 'completeness') can be seen as questionable (Sloane et al., 1985; Yanovski et al., 1992). On the basis of the literature at least, the quality of assessments, judgements and decisions in telephone consultations may not be as high as one might assume.

DECISION SUPPORT FOR TELEPHONE CONSULTATION

It has been suggested that formal protocols/guidelines should be used to improve patient assessment (Evans et al., 1993; Isaacman et al., 1992). Decision support systems are one way in which such protocols or guidelines can be provided. There are broadly two approaches to providing decision support for telephone consultation: an algorithmic (or protocol) driven approach or a guideline based approach. An algorithmic approach provides a structured pathway of questions and answers, systematically prioritising needs and identifying the level of advice that should be given. A guideline based approach is likely to encourage greater flexibility and judgement from the user by providing a structure for the consultation. It provides a series of prompts for assessment and suggested levels of response based on symptoms (Lattimer & Crouch, 1999).

Several studies report the use of protocols in the form of binary decision algorithms (branching decision trees directing the flow of questions based on yes/no responses) in the assessment of patients during face to face triage (Berman et al., 1989; Brillman et al., 1996; Slay & Riskin, 1976; Wilson et al., 1981) and in telephone triage (Levy et al., 1979; Strasser et al., 1979; Wachter et al., 1999). An example of a system using a guideline approach is the Telephone Advice System (TAS) (Crouch, 2000; Crouch et al., 1996b). This system is based on a cognitive model of assessment and decision making designed to reflect and augment nurses' natural assessment and decision making processes.

Protocol or algorithmic approaches

A number of studies have explored the use and effectiveness of protocol/ algorithmic approaches to decision support. Levy et al. (1979) describe the development and field testing of 28 protocols for paediatric triage in both a Health Maintenance Organisation (HMO) and an Emergency Department in the US. Two clinical assistants applied the protocols over the phone. In both settings there was a higher referral rate to hospital facilities than judged necessary by a clinical panel (Levy et al., 1979). Berman et al. (1989) evaluated a computer based binary algorithm system used by assistants in an emergency department. A retriage rate of 1.26% was identified, indicating high sensitivity (98.7%). Specificity was not determined because a false positive rate for one of the arms of the trial was not measured. Berman et al. (1989) conclude that computer guided protocols used by minimally qualified individuals are effective. Strasser et al. (1979) conducted a controlled clinical trial of health assistants providing telephone triage calls in a large emergency department. There was a 16% difference between groups in terms of referral to hospital, with the treatment group (using the protocols) referring more children to hospital than the control group (consisting of physicians and nurses). However, the researchers – using questions taken from nationally recognised guidelines to examine the content of the consultations – identified deficiencies in the assessments made by the control group. In the control group of 76 calls concerning upper respiratory tract infections (URTIs), there was no mention of fever (19%), duration of symptoms (21%), age (11%) and, in 79% of cases, the presence of other medical problems.

Considerable variation in practice has been noticed between physician, nurse and computer based triage. Brillman et al. (1996) compared triage by non-qualified clinicians with that by nurses and physicians and found considerable variation between the three groups. There was greater agreement between physician and nurse triage than between physician and computer software. Considerable variation in the approach to triage was identified. The physician, although given the opportunity, did not examine the patient but rather made their decision on the basis of a review of the nurse documentation. Similarly, the crossover nature of the design could have exposed the patient to the types of questions they were likely to be asked the second time leading to earlier disclosure of salient information.

The literature reviewed earlier in this chapter has identified weaknesses in the assessment process during telephone consultation. Greater consistency in terms of triage decision making has been demonstrated with non-qualified clinicians using binary algorithm protocols. However, the trials of the protocols have been limited to the sites of their development (host sites). When the same protocol systems have been evaluated in other sites, the results have not been so favourable. An example is the evaluation of the AMOS system (Berman et al., 1989). In a site other than the host site, significant differences were observed and inappropriate and/or excessive triaging (Brillman et al., 1996) was the result. It seems likely that the exportability of computer based protocols is questionable.

Limitations of the protocol or algorithmic approach

Farrand et al. (1995) found considerable resistance to formalising nurse's decision making in the Emergency Medical Services (EMS) system in Montreal. They identified a tendency for professional judgement to override decision support tools that did not allow flexible processing of information provided spontaneously by the callers. They also found that the choice of a single protocol for each call felt unnatural to professionals. Often clinicians would spontaneously integrate, in parallel, multiple aspects of a problem. When attempting to formalise nurses' decision making processes using artificial intelligence, the complexity of the decision making process was revealed. Analysis of the accuracy of the decision making using an expert panel and review of 1006 calls revealed almost perfect sensitivity with telephone triage (decision whether to send EMS resources or not) and specificity rates of 0.55. The researchers found that there was a necessary compromise between sensitivity and specificity in different cases and that decision times were related to the urgency of the call – results that suggest that professional nurses utilise sophisticated judgement processes (Farrand et al., 1995).

These findings have been confirmed in a recent simulation study of nurse utilisation and compliance with protocols for telephone advice. Wachter et al. (1999) found considerable variation in protocol selection between nurses when presented with the same cases and poor interrater reliability in the final advice offered. There were differences in protocol selection, with an average of three different protocols being used by nurses to make a disposition in each case. In one case (asthma) where all the nurses used the same protocol to arrive at a disposition, the 12 nurses reached four different end points. The findings of this study do not support the assumption that protocols result in standardisation, indeed the results of Watcher et al.'s study (1999) indicate that 'nurses did not reliably choose the same protocol in a given case and did not reach the same triage endpoint even when they followed the same protocol'. This study was experimental, using actors to play the part of patients with the cases being delivered to nurses in their own homes, and so the ecological validity of the simulation is questionable. However, it could be argued that the assessments and judgements were being conducted under optimal conditions, without the pressures of time and other responsibilities.

The constricting nature of protocols on professional assessment and judgement, alluded to by Farrand et al. (1995), is also supported by the post-triage questions asked by Wachter et al. (1999). In the latter's study, 58% of the nurses described feeling confined by the protocols, and that in half of the consultations they believed protocols forced them to focus on irrelevant information. Deviation from protocols was not uncommon, with 42% of nurses admitting to deviating at least once from the protocols during the consultation (Wachter et al., 1999). It appears that nurses are reluctant to override professional judgement just to follow protocols (Poole et al., 1993; Wachter et al., 1999).

An alternative approach using a cognitive model of decision making (the TAS model)

The nature of telephone consultation and the limitations of existing approaches to decision support represent an opportunity for the development of an alternative approach to providing decision support. The TAS system (Crouch, 2000; Crouch et al., 1996a) is based on a cognitive model of assessment and decision making and mirrors real life approaches to nurses' assessment, judgement and decision making. The following sections will outline the theoretical model, software development and testing.

Development of the TAS model: knowledge elicitation

The development of the model involved eliciting 'expert' knowledge of cognitive processes during telephone assessment and advice and checking that the model was representative of a larger group of emergency nurses. This knowledge was to form the basic structure for modelling the cognitive processes embodied in the decision support program. Knowledge elicitation was undertaken in two broad areas: the development of the cognitive model to be embodied in the computer software and obtaining the clinical information that forms the knowledge base of the software.

There were several stages to the knowledge elicitation process, including structured observation of practice, introspection and forward scenario planning, and diagrammatic representation of the cognitive processes using hypothetical telephone calls. A fuller explanation of these approaches can be found in Box 10.4.

Box 10.4 Approaches to knowledge elicitation

◆ *Structured observation of practice in the form of active participation on behalf of the elicitor and expert* (Cooke, 1994)* – observation is normally a passive exercise. Given the nature of telephone consultation, observation of those consulting would have revealed little of their cognitive processes. Active participation in telephone consultation, whilst recording observations of the process was therefore employed. Thought processes during telephone consultations were noted down.

◆ *Introspection and forward scenario simulation to focus on the cognitive processes (by both the elicitor and expert)* – this process made use of a simulation of cases; the elicitor provided details of the initial situation, the expert then talked through the problem solving in the case, identifying his or her thoughts whilst solving the problem.

◆ *Diagrammatic representations of hypothetical consultations drawn to map the assessment and decision points for a number of scenarios (by the elicitor) (Cooke, 1994)* – the calls described above were mapped onto paper to diagrammatically present the steps in the process of assessment and decision making.

---

*The elicitor of knowledge (the author) was also one of the experts, having a clinical accident and emergency (A&E) background with a high level of domain specific knowledge. The second expert was also a senior A&E nurse.

Information from these processes was collected in note form. These notes were brought together and discussed by the elicitor and expert. Common themes were apparent between the notes taken from the actual calls and those identified in the scenario simulations. These themes or occurrences were recorded and formed the basis of the cognitive model. Structured exploratory interviews were then conducted with three A&E nurses experienced in telephone consultation to confirm the findings of the elicitor and expert (Cooke, 1994).

Using the methods of knowledge elicitation and the data from the exploratory interviews, a cognitive model of decision making during telephone consultation was developed. The broad components of the cognitive model are presented in Box 10.5.

Although this model is presented in terms of input, process and outcome, not all of the elements described will occur in every consultation. Nor will they occur sequentially, because key factors such as presenting symptoms or duration of complaint can influence a decision to go straight to outcome, with very little time spent on gathering additional input.

Level of decision support

Given the perceived deficiencies in assessment, the computer based decision support system was designed to assist in data gathering and information

---

Box 10.5 The TAS cognitive model

Input

◆ elicitation of reason for call
◆ consideration of patient stated problem.

Process

◆ confirmatory questioning
◆ hypothesis generation
◆ alternative hypothesis exploration
◆ identification of causal markers (answers or related symptoms, influencing decision making).

Outcome

◆ confirmatory questions to back up decision
◆ relaying outcome and advice
◆ negotiation
◆ close of consultation with caveat (call back if problem deteriorates).

matching. The program was designed to embody the input, process and outcome elements of the cognitive model. The level of decision support was intended to structure and systematise the assessment of patients, to provide a framework of assessment prompts and to suggest levels of urgency based on presenting complaints or symptoms.

The clinical knowledge base of the software was developed through expert opinion, current research, clinical textbooks and manuals. The range of clinical topics was identified through exploratory work on demand for telephone advice (Crouch et al., 1996b; Dale et al., 1995), a survey of local practice nurses (Williams et al., 1995), exploration of staff views of developing telephone advice in the A&E department (Dale et al., 1995) and through a review of the literature on calls made to emergency and primary care centres (Egleston et al., 1994; Kernohan et al., 1992; Molyneux et al., 1994; Singh et al., 1991).

The software in practice

The software was piloted in a number of clinical settings and the system was seen to be reliable, safe and acceptable (Crouch et al., 1996a). The safety and effectiveness of the system has been evaluated independently in a randomised controlled trial (Lattimer et al., 1998), the results of which indicate that the model of nurse telephone triage supported by the decision support software (TAS) is safe and led to a significant reduction in GP workload. Similar benefits have been observed in a recent study of callers to a GP surgery requesting a same day consultation (Vorster, 1999).

The effect of the software was explored using an experimental study with 16 A&E nurses. The nurses were allocated to either an experimental or control group; the experimental group used the decision support software and the control group continued with their normal practice. Actors presented five simulated cases representing calls normally received in A&E to the nurses in the study. The ecological validity of the cases (that is the extent to which they reflect real life) was established using a panel of A&E clinicians (Crouch, 2000). Using an instrument developed through a Delphi study to establish the completeness of the assessment of the simulated cases, the effect of the system on the assessments was explored. This resulted in a significant change in practice with the introduction of decision support software. Nurses who consulted using the software conducted more clinically adequate and complete assessments than those who did not. An associated change in length of consultation was also observed with the experimental group when decision support was used.

The increase in consultation length was associated with the increase in the depth of the assessment.

Consultation style was also affected using the decision support software, with a focus on less open questions and an increase in closed questions. Significantly more information was elicited using this approach (Crouch, 2000). A trend towards recommending a less urgent form of health care was also seen with those nurses using the decision support software. The effect of the system on cognitive processes used during telephone consultation was also explored; it appears that the use of decision support software in consultations alters the cognitive processing of the nurses during the consultation. A possible explanation being that a resequencing of cognitive operators used in the problem solving task occurs. It is also possible that the framework of operators or clinical cues acts as a compensatory mechanism for the loss of visual cues during telephone consultation. However, further research is required to ascertain the actual effect of the software on assimilation of information during decision making (Crouch, 2000). It appears that the use of computer based decision support software may enhance the clinical safety of telephone consultation by preventing the premature closure of consultations highlighted earlier.

NHS DIRECT

Perhaps the largest application of decision support software in the NHS is NHS Direct, the 24 hour nurse led telephone advice service. The fundamental priniciple of NHS Direct is to provide 'easier and faster advice and information for people about health, illness and the NHS so that they are better able to care for themselves and their families' (Department of Health, 1998). The service is configured to receive calls from the general public 24 hours a day about any health related matter. Call handlers (non-professionals) and nurses accept calls from the general public. Using a computer based decision support program they assess the severity of the callers problem, decide the urgency with which they need further health care intervention (or if they can manage the problem at home) and give standardised advice for the caller to follow. Early evaluation of the service shows high levels of caller satisfaction and that the service is safe. The service was established in 1998 and no large scale evaluation of the acceptability of the decision support software to the nurses delivering the service has yet been conducted.

THE FUTURE ROLE OF DECISION SUPPORT FOR NURSING

The provision of health care is changing rapidly in the UK and there has been a recent expansion of nursing roles. With this expansion has come a greater focus on the quality and consistency of care provided, brought together under the guise of clinical governance. Although this chapter has focused on one area of nursing in particular, it is likely that we will see the development of computer based decision support in many areas of nursing in the next decade. Take, for instance, the assessment of a patient in a ward based environment. It is conceivable that the assessment data entered by the nurse, including physiological, biochemical and social factors, would be used to develop a pathway of care. This pathway would be individually tailored but would draw on the knowledge base within the system of patients of a similar age and sex and with similar presenting complaints. This data, together with the current patient profile, would help to identify potential problems for that individual. This would be care planning in real time. Is there a need for a nurse you might ask? The answer has to be yes, because the nurse is a fundamental part of that knowledge base and the system should be supportive rather than directive. The challenge for nursing is to identify the areas of practice where decision support will be of most benefit and to ensure that the design reflects, as near as possible, normal patterns of decision making and augments rather than replaces these processes.

CONCLUSION

This chapter has outlined the principles and some of the approaches given to the provision of computer based decision support. The area of telephone consultation has been taken as an example where decision support, to improve the depth and accuracy of patient assessment, judgement and decision making, has been identified and evaluated. The chapter has also highlighted areas where decision support is likely to play an important part in nursing practice. With the increasing complexity of health care delivery, the emphasis on evidence based practice and the increasingly litigious nature of health care, more effective ways of managing knowledge and improving the safety of care delivery are needed. Computer based decision support provides one source of support. However, such support systems should be clinically not technologically driven and, before widespread adoption, should be formally evaluated.

QUESTIONS FOR DISCUSSION

◆ Are there areas of your clinical practice where you should assess the accuracy of assessment, judgement and decision making?

◆ How could you do this?

◆ How could decision support software enhance these processes?

ANNOTATED FURTHER READING

Deutsch, T., Carson, E., & Ludwig, E. (1994). *Dealing with medical knowledge: Computers in clinical decision making.* New York: Plenum Press.

A great (although not always simple) introduction to the anatomy of medical and health care decisions and the principles, practice and theory of computerised decision support.

Johnston, M.E., Langton, K.B., Haynes, R.B., & Mathieu, A. (1994). Effects of computer-based clinical decision support systems on clinician performance and patient outcome. A critical appraisal of research. *Annals of Internal Medicine, 120*(2), 135–142.

A comprehensive review of the impact of decision support technology on medical decision making (much of which is relevant to nurses).

REFERENCES

Aitken, M.E., Carey, M.J., & Kool, B. (1995). Telephone advice about an infant given by after-hours clinics and emergency departments. *New Zealand Medical Journal, 108*, 315–317.

Berman, D.A., Coleridge, S.T., & McMurray, T.A. (1989). Computerized algorithm directed triage in the emergency department. *Annals of Emergency Medicine, 18*(2), 141–144.

Brillman, J.C., Doezema, D., Tandberg, D. et al. (1996). Triage: Limitations in predicting need for emergent care and hospital admissions. *Annals of Emergency Medicine, 27*(4), 493–500.

Brown, S.B. & Eberle, B.J. (1974). Use of the telephone by pediatric house staff: A technique for pediatric care not taught. *The Journal of Pediatrics, 84*(1), 117–119.

Buchanan, B.G. & Shortliffe, E.H. (1985). *Rule-based expert systems – the MYCIN experiments of the Stanford heuristics programming project.* Massachusetts: Addison-Wesley.

Clancey, W.J. & Shortliffe, E.H. (1984). Medical artificial intelligence programs. In: Clancey, W.J. & Shortliffe, E.H. (eds), *Readings in medical artificial intelligence – the first decade.* Massachusetts: Addison-Wesley.

Cooke, N.J. (1994). Varieties of knowledge elicitation techniques. *International Journal of Human–Computer Studies, 41*, 801–849.

Crouch, R. (2000). *An investigation into the effects of a computer based decision support program on accident and emergency nurses' assessment strategies in telephone consultation.* Guildford: PhD Thesis, University of Surrey.

Crouch, R., Patel, A., & Dale, J. (1996a). Paediatric calls to an inner city A&E department: service demand and advice given. *Accident and Emergency Nursing, 4*, 170–174.

Crouch, R., Patel, A., Williams, S., & Dale, J. (1996b). An analysis of telephone calls to an inner-city accident and emergency department. *Journal of the Royal Society of Medicine, 89,* 324–328.

Dale, J., Williams, S., & Crouch, R. (1995). Development of telephone advice in accident and emergency: establishing the views of the staff. *Nursing Standard, 9*(21), 28–31.

de Dombal, F.T. (1988). Computer-aided diagnosis of acute abdominal pain: the British experience. In: Dowie, J. & Elstein, A. (eds), *Professional judgment: A reader in clinical decision making.* Cambridge: Cambridge University Press.

de Dombal, F.T., Leaper, D.J., Staniland, J.R. et al. (1972). Computer-aided diagnosis of acute abdominal pain. *British Medical Journal, 2,* 9–13.

Department of Health (1998). A first class service. London: The Stationery Office.

Dowie, J. (1993). Clinical decision analysis: Background and introduction. In: Llewelyn, H. & Hopkins, A. (eds), *Analysing how we reach clinical decisions.* London: Royal College of Physicians.

Dowie, J. & Elstein, A. (1988). *Professional judgement. A reader in clinical decision making.* Cambridge: Cambridge University Press.

Duda, R.O. & Shortliffe, E.H. (1983). Expert systems research. *Science, 220,* 261–268.

Egleston, C.V., Kelly, H.C., & Cope, A.R. (1994). Use of a telephone advice line in an accident and emergency department. *British Medical Journal, 308,* 31.

Evans, R.J., Mccabe, M., Allen, H., Rainer, T., & Richmond, P.W. (1993). Telephone advice in the accident and emergency department: A survey of current practice. *Archives of Emergency Medicine, 10,* 216–219.

Farrand, L., Leprohon, J., Kalina, M., Champagne, F., Contandriopoulos, A.P., & Preker, A. (1995). The role of protocols and professional judgement in emergency medical dispatching. *European Journal of Emergency Medicine, 2*(3), 136–148.

Fox, J. (1993). Decision-support systems as safety-critical components: Towards a safety culture for medical informatics (Editorial). *Methods of Information in Medicine, 32,* 345–348.

Greer, M.L. (1992). RXPERT: A prototype expert system for formulary decision making. *The Annals of Pharmacotherapy, 26,* 2444–2450.

Greitzer, L., Stapleton, F.B., Wright, L., & Wedgewood, R.J. (1976). Telephone assessment of illness by practicing physicians. *The Journal of Pediatrics, 88,* 880–882.

Heathfield, H.A. & Wyatt, J. (1993). Philosophies for the design and development of clinical decision support systems. *Methods of Information in Medicine, 32,* 1–8.

Isaacman, D.J., Verdile, V.P., Kohen, F.P., & Verdile, L.A. (1992). Pediatric telephone advice in the emergency department: Results of a mock scenario. *Pediatrics, 89*(1), 35–39.

Kernohan, S.M., Moir, P.A., & Beattie, T.F. (1992). Telephone calls to a paediatric accident and emergency department. *Health Bulletin, 50*(3), 233–236.

Koch, B. & McGovern, J. (1993). EXTEND: A protype expert system for teaching nursing diagnosis. *Computers in Nursing, 11*(1), 35–41.

Lattimer, V. & Crouch, R. (1999). Nurse telephone consultation. In: Salisbury, S., Dale, J. & Hallam, L. (eds), *24 hour primary care.* Oxford: Radcliffe Medical Press.

Levy, J.C., Rosekrans, J., Lamb, A., Friedman, M., Kaplan, D., & Stasser, P. (1979). Development and field testing of protocols for the management of pediatric telephone calls: Protocols for pediatric telephone calls. *Pediatrics, 64*(5), 558–563.

Luker, K.A. & Caress, A. (1992). Evaluating computer assisted learning for renal patients. *International Journal of Nursing Studies, 29*(3), 237–250.

Molyneux, E., Jones, N., Aldom, G., & Molyneux, B. (1994). Audit of telephone advice in a paediatric accident and emergency department. *Journal of Accident and Emergency Medicine, 11,* 246–249.

Moreno, H.R. & Plant, R.T. (1993). A prototype decision support system for differential diagnosis of psychotic, mood and organic mental disorders. *Medical Decision Making, 13,* 43–48.

Ott, J.E., Bellaire, J., Machotka, P., & Moon, J.B. (1974). Patient management by telephone by child health associates and pediatric house officers. *Journal of Medical Education, 49,* 596–600.

Perrin, E.C. & Goodman, H.C. (1978). Telephone management of acute pediatric illness. *The New England Journal of Medicine, 298*(3), 130–135.

Poole, S.R., Schmitt, B.D., Carruth, T., Peterson-Smith, A., & Slusarski, M. (1993). After-hours coverage: An application of area-wide telephone triage and advice system for paediatric practices. *Pediatrics, 92,* 670–679.

Shortliffe, E.H. (1976). *Computer based medical consultations: MYCIN.* New York: Elsevier.

Shortliffe, E.H. (1990). Clinical decision-support systems. In: Shortliffe, E.H. & Perreault, L.E. (eds), *Medical informatics: Computer applications in health care.* Massachusetts: Addison-Wesley.

Singh, G., Barton, D., & Bodiwala, G.G. (1991). Accident and emergency department's response to patients' enquiries by telephone. *Journal of the Royal Society of Medicine, 84*, 345–346.

Slay, L.E. & Riskin, W.G. (1976). Algorithm directed triage in an emergency department. *JACEP, 5*, 8669–8876.

Sloane, P.D., Egelhoff, C., Curtis, P., McGaghie, W., & Evens, S. (1985). Physician decision making over the telephone. *The Journal of Family Practice, 21*(4), 279–284.

Strasser, P.H., Levy, J.C., Lamb, G.A., & Rosekrans, J. (1979). Controlled clinical trial of pediatric telephone protocols. *Pediatrics, 64*(5), 553–557.

Verdaguer, A., Patak, A., Sancho, J.J., Sierra, C., & Sanz, F. (1992). Validation of the medical expert system PNEUMON-IA. *Computer and Biomedical Research, 25*, 511–526.

Verdile, V.P., Paris, P.M., Stewart, R.D., & Verdile, L.A. (1989). Emergency department telephone advice. *Annals of Emergency Medicine, 18*, 278–282.

Vorster, M. (1999). Behind the lines. *Health Service Journal, 109*(5655), 24–25.

Wachter, D.A., Brillman, J.C., Lewis, J., & Sapien, R.E. (1999). Pediatric telephone triage protocols: Standard decision making or a false sense of security. *Annals of Emergency Medicine, 33*(4), 388–394.

Williams, S., Crouch, R., & Dale, J. (1995). Providing health-care advice by telephone. *Professional Nurse, 10*(12), 750–752.

Wilson, L.O., Wilson, F.P., & Wheeler, M. (1981). Computerized triage of pediatric patients: Automated triage algorithms. *Annals of Emergency Medicine, 10*(12), 636–640.

Wyatt, J. (1991). Computer-based knowledge systems. *The Lancet, 338*, 1431–1436.

Wyatt, J. & Spiegelhalter, D. (1990). Evaluating medical expert systems: What to test and why? *Medical Informatics, 15*(3), 205–217.

Yanovski, S.Z., Yanovski, J.A., Malley, J.D., Brown, R.L., & Balaban, D.J. (1992). Telephone triage by primary care physicians. *Pediatrics, 89*(4), 701–706.

Zielstorff, R.D., Barnett, G.O., Fitzmaurice, J.B. et al. (1994). A decision support system for troubleshooting pulmonary artery catheter waveforms. In: Grobe, S.J. & Plyuyter-Wenting, E.S.P. (eds), *Nursing informatics: An international overview for nursing in a technological era.* Amsterdam: Elsevier.

11

Decision making and judgement in nursing – some conclusions

Dawn Dowding   Carl Thompson

This chapter pulls together the 'take home messages' from this book. We did not set out to – nor have we delivered – a definitive 'how to' guide for judgement and decision making. Rather, this text is an introduction to some of the key arguments, research evidence and clinical examples appertaining to clinical judgement and decision making. If this is the first time that you have encountered this body of work, we hope that the arguments we have highlighted and the resources that accompany each chapter will be your entry to an exciting (and fruitful) area of research inquiry and practice development. If you are more *au fait* with the literature, research and arguments we have drawn on, we hope that you will pick up the academic baton and use some of the material in teaching, practice development and efforts to improve the decisions you and your colleagues make.

KEY ISSUES

◆ This book has examined many of the issues associated with researching and with developing judgement and clinical decision making in nursing and midwifery practice. It has described how individuals make decisions and judgements in practice, the nature of the decisions and judgements nurses face and ways of making sense of uncertain information (clinical, research or cognitive), and has introduced techniques and technologies for supporting decisions and judgements. All of these areas of scrutiny were chosen for examination in this book because we wanted to generate practical, clinically relevant messages for clinicians and researchers. This book is intended to act as the basis for practical developments, as opposed to esoteric, academic exercises with little or no relevance to clinicians and managers delivering (and supporting the delivery of) health care.

A STARTING POINT: UNDERSTANDING THE NATURE OF THE DECISIONS WE MAKE IN PRACTICE

A message we hope you take away from this book is the importance of examining your own practice. Health care practitioners need to have a good understanding of the types of judgements and decisions they make in practice, together with the information used to inform these.

Regarding judgements, Chapter 3 highlights that one of the main focuses of nursing practice is assessment. However, assessment is not an end in itself. If assessment is treated as a standalone area of nursing activity then it rapidly becomes meaningless. Assessment – as a process – is intricately linked to healthcare decision making. As a practitioner, you need to be aware of the judgements made during the assessment process (and how accurate – or not – they may be). If judgements are made on the basis of information, gathered during assessment, which is incomplete, redundant or inaccurate then resulting decision choices will always be flawed, or at the very least prone to errors. At a number of key points in this book we have striven to show how asking the simple questions 'Why am I carrying out this assessment? How accurate are the tools, tests and questions I am using? And how will I use the results?' can pay dividends.

As well as locating processes such as assessment in the context of clinical judgement, Dorothy McCaughan in Chapter 6 illustrated the importance of understanding the types of decisions nurses make in practice. All decisions in health care have an element of uncertainty attached. By understanding the kinds of decisions you make (diagnostic, treatment or intervention selection, communicating risks or harm) you are better able to gain a purchase on the appropriate sorts of evidence with which to address associated uncertainties. Understanding decisions made in practice is the foundation for an evidence based approach to practice (from decisions flow clinical questions and systematic search strategies). Moreover, when you understand the nature of the decisions you face you are better able to take advantage of the wealth of decision support strategies available to clinicians – both strategic (such as decision analysis) and computerised.

EVIDENCE BASED PRACTICE – SYSTEMATICALLY PLANNING ACTION FOR HEALTHCARE DECISION MAKING

In Chapter 7, Flemming and Fenton provided an overview of the systematic process for reliably filling the information gaps that arise in practice. As well as offering a strategy for meeting individual information needs and improving decisions, an evidence based approach to practice offers a common language and set of ideas to which many professionals (from all disciplines) are signing up. The language and core ideas provide a form of currency for negotiation in the process of introducing clinical change. Similarly, it is becoming increasingly clear that advances in the science (and art) of searching for research evidence, formulating clinical questions, critical appraisal and implementation, are just as relevant to nurses as other disciplines. It is our belief that this approach encourages the delivery of health care by clinical teams and discourages unidisciplinary, narrow and ill informed attempts to change professional practice.

'JUGGLING JELLY' – TRACKING AND HANDLING THE INFORMATION THAT FEEDS DECISION MAKING AND JUDGEMENT

Of course, any systematic approach of giving due weight to the information generated through research, clinical expertise, economic reality and listening to the patient will only be as good as the information the clinician is faced with. The information that impacts on decision making is complex, often combining qualitative and quantitative characteristics, often emotive and sometimes conflicting. Handling such a mixed bag of data, and knowing which messages should carry the most weight, is covered (in varying degrees) in Chapters 2, 3 and 4.

In the absence of accurate tests for ascertaining the probability of someone developing a pressure sore, or the accuracy of a routine screening device such as urinalysis, the clinician's best guide to the likelihood of a complication or disease (and nurses will increasingly be asked to diagnose disease) is good baseline data (e.g. the prevalence of a disease in the population you work with). Such information needs can be filled in part by good quality research evidence but we hope that this book will encourage you to link your clinical audit, governance and decision making activity so that clinical questions, appraised evidence and quality data on local prevalence of common conditions are all linked. One of the most useful things you could start doing is collecting prevalence data in your practice area (such as pressure sore rates, rates of infection post urinary catheterisation, numbers of venous leg ulcers). This kind of data is important for assessing the effectiveness of clinical tests (where such tests exist) but is equally important as a way of identifying common problems in your patient population, as well as indicating ways changes in practice may affect the outcomes of care.

Chapters 2, 3, 4 and 7 also highlight the fact that research evidence is not the only source of information health care practitioners use to inform their practice. Moreover, we unequivocally reject the normative principle idea that it ever should be. However, prevalence data does provide reliable prior probabilities of a particular condition or problem arising in your patient population. When combined with information on the accuracy of a diagnostic test or the effectiveness of a particular intervention, then such information becomes increasingly useful. When combined with a clinician's experience, the preferences of the patient and a portfolio of evidence based resources, then such information is not only useful but increasingly powerful. What Chapters 2, 3 and 4 illustrate is that perhaps some of the weight we attach to intuitive feelings of 'correctness' or a sense of 'blind' logic need redressing.

BUILDING YOUR OWN COGNITIVE TOOLKIT – DEVELOPING THE SKILLS FOR IMPROVING DECISION MAKING AND JUDGEMENT

Different kinds of decision merit (and generate) different kinds of information, which in turn require different processing techniques during decision making. A number of the chapters offer practical hints and tips to help improve your decision making and avoid some of the pitfalls associated with the ways human beings process information. These hints and tips constitute a fairly generic 'toolkit' and all focus on the idea that reducing the errors associated with clinical practice is a good thing. What the chapters do not do is prescribe the amounts of weight you should attach to information for specific decisions. Indeed, this would be impossible, given the highly individualised nature of clinical decision making and the infinite combinations of resources, research evidence, clinical expertise and patient preference associated with just one clinician's daily workload.

The lens model discussed in Chapter 5 (associated with the social judgement approach to judgement and decision making) provides a way of capturing or attaching importance to information in both the ecological and the judgement situation. This provides a more explicit picture of what the balance of information use should, or does, look like in practice. Clearly, such an approach represents a significant departure from merely describing decision making, towards providing a framework for prescribing how decisions should be made.

Chapter 4 highlights the discrepancy between descriptive approaches to decision making (what individuals do in practice) and normative approaches (what they should do for optimal decision making). Offredy's work illustrates that, in reality, health care professionals are really doing a bit of both. The fact that people do not act as linear information processing machines is the basis for a raft of 'real life' decision making theoretical frameworks and support technologies, perhaps the most influential of which are based on the ideas of the eighteenth century cleric, Thomas Bayes.

Textbook ways of teaching diagnosis tend towards the axiom 'given disease X, what is the probability of exhibiting symptoms Y and Z?'. However, in reality most practitioners reason according to the (subtly different) formula of 'given the symptoms Y and Z, what is the probability of having disease *X?'*. Bayesian approaches to decision making take as their starting point these real life ways in which human beings process information. Bayesian decision support technologies, such as the DIAGNOSTICA (Blinowska et al., 1993) system for helping decide whether a patient has secondary or essential hypertension, are all based on this kind of reasoning. The importance of understanding Bayesian approaches to techniques such as decision analysis are that they offer more accurate means of revising the *a posteriori* probabilities uncovered by your consideration of the available research evidence and your patient's preferences. In depth discussion of the field of Bayesian decision theory lies outside the scope of this text but readers are strongly encouraged to acquaint themselves with the ideas and techniques of this important area if they are considering developing or exploring decision support further.

HARNESSING TECHNOLOGY

In the final part of the book the focus moves away from generic techniques for systematically addressing how information is used to inform decision making towards the use of formal systems for supporting decision making.

Practice guidelines offer a relatively flexible way of ensuring that relevant key decision points incorporate lessons learned from good quality research evidence. Guidelines encourage nurses to address key decision points and revise their assessments of the likelihood of problems, outcomes or decision end points. In conjunction with other change initiatives, such as continuing professional development, audit, feedback, and a thorough diagnosis of the likely barriers to change in clinical settings, they can be a powerful mechanism for changing professional practice (Thomas et al., 1999).

Guidelines, if used clumsily, can sometimes be interpreted as rigid protocols. Obviously, such rigidity in interpretation is misguided; as has already been highlighted, a good decision is one that recognises the individuality of patient circumstance and preference, and the limitations of one's own expertise and resource availability.

Decision analysis takes the idea of decision support systems one stage further. The technique is under utilised in nursing (perhaps because nurse researchers have only recently begun to explore the kinds of decisions the profession makes). We believe that decision analysis offers a real challenge for disseminators of research evidence and for those in practice development. The technique has enormous potential for making the choices associated with practice more transparent, both to other health care practitioners and to patients. In areas such as wound care, asthma and diabetes, where diagnosis and treatment selection are increasingly becoming part of the nurse's role, then the role of decision analysis in nurse decision making could be developed and evaluated.

It would be a foolish commentator, however, who denied that decision analytic techniques, Bayesian approaches to diagnosis and policy capturing model construction, do not incur extensive opportunity costs (especially time). In the twenty-first century, however, increases in computing power and portability, as well as the expansion of the science of health informatics, mean that such 'tried and tested' techniques could become less unwieldy to use in practice. In Chapter 10, Robert Crouch discusses the use of computerised decision support systems in nursing. With the increasing role of information technology in all walks of life, this is obviously an important and timely issue for discussion. What is important to recognise here is that the theoretical and empirical foundations alluded to in the other chapters make such technologies a viable option for practitioners. Evidence based practice, social judgement theory and decision analysis are standalone techniques that do not depend on technology to make them real or usable in practice. However, the technology offered by computer support systems allows these techniques to be more accessible to practitioners, as demonstrated for example by the Cogent project (Eccles et al., 2000). The laborious calculations that are involved in social judgement approaches and decision analysis can be carried out by such systems, leaving practitioners free to concentrate on interpreting and applying the 'bottom line' to clinical practice. These technologies can also ensure that patients benefit directly from the use of technology (e.g. telephone consultations). However, it is important to emphasise that all types of support system (computerised or not) are not a replacement for professional judgement and decision making. Even the most sophisticated instrument can only ever inform decisions – ultimately, professional decision making in health care is a human rather than a technical exercise.

IMPLICATIONS FOR POLICY AND RESEARCH

Evidence based decision making in all areas of healthcare practice is expected to become the norm in the delivery of health services. Clinical governance, the increasing need to demonstrate quality in care and the increasing use of litigation mean that it is imperative that nurses and midwives consider the nature of their clinical judgements and decisions.

Alongside these policy drivers, nursing is continuing its struggle for recognition as a profession with its own knowledge base, specialist characteristics and unique contribution to the production of health. Initiatives such as nurse prescribing and the use of nurse practitioners in general practices (as discussed by Maxine Offredy in Ch. 4) are indicative that at least some of these claims are being given credence by policy makers. However, with a mandate for autonomous professional decision making comes an equal measure of professional responsibility. This responsibility means being able to justify, explain and defend the judgements and decisions you make. Hopefully, the tools and techniques that have been discussed in this book will go some way towards helping practitioners fulfil this need.

What we hope we have shown throughout this book is the existence of research literature, often from other disciplines, which can be used to inform judgement and decision making practice in nursing and midwifery. However, there is still a large amount of research that needs to be carried out in this area. Until this work is carried out it is difficult to state with any degree of confidence the quality of decisions being made, or to promote specific strategies for delivering optimal decision choices. In particular we still need to identify:

◆ The judgements and decisions nurses and midwives are making in a number of areas of clinical practice. This baseline data will help in the development of evidence based solutions to clinical problems. Some initial work has been carried out in acute and primary care (Thompson et al., 2000) but more is needed.
◆ The quality of nursing judgements and decisions. How accurate are the judgements we make? The predictions offered to patients? How effective are the treatment solutions we consider? Clinical governance and the evidence based climate of practice and policy will make the generation of answers to such questions ever more important.
◆ Ways of assisting practitioners in their judgement and decision making. Much of the literature on research dissemination has shown categorically that just providing research evidence for passive consumption by clinicians does not change practice. We need to consider how we can assist practitioners to incorporate this evidence into their decision making in ways that are usable and flexible enough to cope with the dynamic nature of health care. Decision support systems may well be the way forward. However, this research also needs to consider the impact that such systems have on patient outcomes.

This book has striven to provide background material for those considering the improvement of their decision making, designing or conducting research in this area, or simply addressing a hitherto neglected area of practice development. We hope that you enjoy your journey into the fascinating area of clinical decision making and judgement in nursing. Moreover, we hope that the book has provided as many questions as answers.

REFERENCES

Blinowska, A., Chatellier, G., Wojtasik, J., & Bernier, B. (1993). DIAGNOSTICA: A Bayesian diagnostic decision aid applied to hypertension. *IEEE Transactions on Biomedical Engineering, 40*, 230–237.

Eccles, M., Grimshaw, J., Steen, N. et al. (2000). The design and analysis of a randomised controlled trial to evaluate computerised decision support in primary care: The COGENT study. *Family Practice, 17*, 180–186.

Thomas, L., McColl, E., Cullum, N., Rousseau, N., & Soutter, J. (1999). Clinical guidelines in nursing, midwifery and the therapies: A systematic review. *Journal of Advanced Nursing, 30*(1), 40–50.

Thompson, C., McCaughan, D., Cullum, N., Sheldon, T.A., Thompson, D.R., & Mulhall, A. (2000). *Nurses' use of research information in clinical decision making: A descriptive and analytical study – final report.* London: The National Co-ordinating Centre for Service Delivery and Organisation, NHS R&D Programme.

Index